Dear God, Why Can't
We Have a Baby

Dear God, Why Can't We Have a Baby?

A Guide for the Infertile Couple

**John and Sylvia Van Regenmorter
and Joe S. McIlhaney Jr., M.D.**

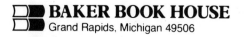
BAKER BOOK HOUSE
Grand Rapids, Michigan 49506

Much of the commentary by Dr. Joe S. McIlhaney, Jr., is taken from chapter 11 of *1250 Health-Care Questions Women Ask*, copyright 1985 by Baker Book House. The comments are in bolder type with a ragged left margin, except for chapter 3 which is adapted from Dr. McIlhaney's material. Most of the glossary items were also written by Dr. McIlhaney.

Scripture quotations not otherwise marked are from the Holy Bible, New International Version. Copyright 1973, 1978, 1984 by International Bible Society. Used by permission of Zondervan Bible Publishers. The quotation from The Living Bible, © 1971 is used with permission of Tyndale House Publishers.

The authors wish to express appreciation to the following for permission to quote copyrighted material:

Augsburg Publishing House, for use of excerpts from *The Wedded Unmother* by Kay Halverson with Karen Ness and *Coping with Infertility* by Judith A. Stigger. Christianity Today for use of excerpts from "Other Views on Embryo Transfer" by Lewis Smedes and "Embryo Transfer: A Woman Can Now Give Birth to Her Own Stepchild" by Robert G. Wells. CRC Publications, a Ministry of the Christian Reformed Church, for use of excerpts from articles that appeared in The Banner. E. P. Dutton for use of excerpts from *We Want to Have a Baby* by James T. Howard, Jr., and Dodi Schultz and *You Can Have a Baby* by Sherwin A. Kaufman, M.D. Prentice-Hall for use of excerpts from *Infertility: A Guide for the Childless Couple* by Barbara Eck Menning. Resolve, Inc., for use of excerpts from National Resolve Newsletters. TIME magazine for use of excerpt from "The Baby in the Factory" by Rogert Rosenblatt. Victor Books for use of excerpt from *What Happens When Women Pray* by Evelyn Christiansen. The Zondervan Corporation for use of excerpts from *A Step Further* by Joni Eareckson and Steve Estes and *Where Is God When It Hurts?* by Philip Yancey.

Contents

Introduction   9
1   The Laughter of Little Children   13
2   Avoiding the Early Pitfalls   21
3   What Constitutes a Complete
    Infertility Workup?   35
4   The Infertility Struggle   57
5   Husband vs. Wife or Husband and Wife?   67
6   Beginning to Cope with Infertility   75
7   Family, Friends, and Fellow Christians   85
8   Infertility and the Christian Faith   97
9   What's Right—What's Wrong?   109
10   When Is Enough, Enough?   135
11   Adoption as an Option   139
12   Learning to Live with Infertility   149
    Bibliography   157
    Suggestions for Further Reading   159
    Glossary   161

Introduction

Infertility is the inability to conceive a child or to carry a child to a live birth after one or more years of normal sexual relations. Approximately 10 to 15 percent of the married American population have an infertility problem and the percentages are rising.

Statistics, of course, do not plumb the emotional depth of infertility. Only those couples who have been there, who are part of the 10 to 15 percent, know the pain of infertility for all its worth. We have been there.

Approximately eight years ago we discovered that there was a good possibility we might not have biological children. During the succeeding years we experienced questions: Why, God? We experienced loneliness: Why does everyone around us seem to have children? We experienced well-meaning but ignorant advice: "Why don't you just adopt and you'll get pregnant?" We experienced doubts: Is infertility a curse?

In those years we visited almost half-a-dozen doctors, spent thousands of dollars, and had moments of great expectation quickly crushed by agonizing failure. Through these experiences two things occurred. First, we learned. We learned slowly and sometimes painfully, but we learned.

We learned what we should look for in terms of medical treatment, we learned what to expect by way of ethical questions, we learned what kind of unintended hurts come from loving but ill-advised family and friends, and we learned how to deal with some of the religious doubts that plague many infertile couples.

Secondly, as a Christian couple our desire has grown to share our insights with others who are confronted with infertility.

We wish to acknowledge the contributions of those who helped us write this book. We are grateful to Bev Miller, a fellow traveler down the road of infertility, who provided much encouragement and many insights. To Dr. Ernie Zimbelman, Professor of Counseling at the North American Baptist Seminary, thanks for the discerning advice and for encouraging us toward greater professionalism. Thanks to Dr. Si Lee, a certified reproductive endocrinologist, for helping us analyze some of the medical and ethical problems involved in current infertility treatment. To Pam Jarding, thanks for patiently transforming our messy manuscript into a beautifully typed copy. Thanks, too, to Beth Mulder, a lover of the English language, who helped us care for style and grammar, and to Betty De Vries of Baker Book House for the final editing. They both made us look better than we deserve.

John and Sylvia Van Regenmorter

Introduction

We physicians who provide infertility care continue to see couples who have too long delayed obtaining diagnosis and treatment for their problems. When a couple postpones obtaining care for an infertility problem, that problem will often become so severe that it cannot be corrected, and the couple is subjected to childlessness. It is even more frustrating to have a couple come to us whose infertility care has been delayed by a well-meaning but poorly organized or uninformed physician who has not provided up-to-date care. Unfortunately, the experiences the Van Regenmorters had with such physicians are not unusual.

Hopefully this book will motivate couples who have not been able to achieve pregnancy after twelve months of regular intercourse to consult a doctor who can help them have the biological child they so greatly desire.

Couples who are suffering from infertility can find much help in this book. Books that merely discuss the medical aspects of infertility evaluation and treatment are ignoring the tremendous emotional impact of this problem. Such books also ignore the moral choices faced today by couples with infertility problems. Books that talk only about the emotional stress or the moral dilemmas of infertility are inadequate for properly informing infertile couples. This book discusses the physical, emotional, and moral aspects of infertility and should prove to be satisfying and beneficial in its completeness.

Joe S. McIlhaney, Jr., M.D.

1

The Laughter of Little Children

Sylvia

If it is thy will, grant them the laughter of little children." This was part of a prayer during our marriage ceremony nearly twelve years ago. Little did I realize the number of prayers that would be said and tears that would be shed before we were "granted the laughter of little children."

Looking back, I am rather surprised at myself for assuming all married couples have children. Even though I came from a family of four children, I had an aunt and uncle who were never able to have children. Having close relatives who were childless should have made me realize that having children was not automatically guaranteed, but somehow I assumed I had an inalienable right to be a mother.

Our family spent many summer Saturdays at a nearby Washington lake or the Pacific Ocean with four other families, three of whom had adopted children. The other family had only one child. So I was aware that all married couples did not have biological children but never considered that someday I would be numbered with them.

As I shared these thoughts with John, he told me that he also never gave a thought to not having children. He grew up in a family of six children and he could recall only one couple who were childless.

We assumed that it was indeed God's will for us in time to have children. In fact, within a few months after our marriage, we had already chosen their names: John Mark and Sarah.

About six months after we were married, we left for a one-year internship in the Philippines to assist missionaries in teaching and evangelism. While there we felt a strong urge to adopt a Filipino child because there were many children in that poor nation who needed homes. But we chose to have our biological children first, and then perhaps we would work on adopting a needy Filipino child.

After returning from the Philippines we were most anxious to begin our family. Others obviously were waiting for the same event, since I was frequently asked, "Are you pregnant?" I said "No," but I was sure it wouldn't be long before I could give a very excited "yes" response.

Months passed without a pregnancy occurring, but we did not become alarmed. We were certain that the delay was due to the pressures of recent moves and the challenges of John's new ministry in New Jersey. In the rush of a busy life, a year went by. The fact that I had not conceived was no more than a pinprick in the back of our minds. We did not worry. We did not panic. We felt that God in due time would grace our marriage with children.

Our concern was large enough, however, that we decided to do some reading on the subject of infertility. We found, much to our disappointment, only two books on the topic, both of them written by physicians and quite technical in nature. One of them had been written nearly thirty years earlier.

When two years passed without a pregnancy, we became more concerned. I suggested that I see a doctor. We discussed it quite thoroughly and prayed about it together. The pinprick was beginning to enlarge. I was sure that there was nothing seriously wrong, but wanted to be reassured. I made an appointment with a gynecologist, one who was also an obstetrician. At that point I was not overly concerned that he had expertise in the area of infertility, I simply did not want to change doctors after I became pregnant.

Full of the quiet confidence that many people feel when they finally make the resolution to seek the care of a doctor, I went to keep my appointment. I was relieved when, after what seemed to be a thorough examination, he told me that he could find nothing wrong and that we should simply keep trying. I suggested that perhaps John have a semen analysis and that I begin charting my temperature—that much I had learned from the reading we had done. But the doctor simply said, "Relax, wait six more months, and if nothing happens, come and see me again."

I was naive and did wait several more months, but not six. I was becoming too anxious to let a half-year slip by with no action. Bravely one day I called him and said I would just like him to look at my Basal Body Temperature Chart (BBT chart measures the time of ovulation) and do a semen analysis on John. I was dumbfounded when he said, "I don't really get into infertility work because it is too time consuming. If you are interested in pursuing it, I could suggest another physician." I could have screamed! Why didn't he tell me right from the start? Why didn't he let me know that he would not, probably could not, help me? Why did he keep me anxiously waiting?

I called the recommended physician, only to discover I would have to wait three whole months for an appointment before her schedule and my cycle fit the appointment book. When the day finally came, the receptionist called an hour before my appointment and said, "The doctor is sick today, could you please come in next Thursday instead?" I explained that my cycle would not fit the requirements that had been stressed when I originally called to make my appointment. The receptionist said, "It really doesn't matter." "But why," I asked, "did I initially have to wait three whole months for the right time in my cycle, and now it doesn't matter?" Frustrated and angry, I decided to find another doctor.

I then wrote the American Fertility Society in Atlanta. I was sent the name of a physician in my area whom I decided to call. When I did so, I was informed that she was too busy with obstetric cases to take any new infertility patients.

If I did not hate pregnant women before, I was beginning to now. Not only could they get pregnant, it also seemed that everyone was working for them as well. Didn't anyone care about me, us?

I called the local medical association. They were very friendly but unhelpful. They only referred me to the doctors I had already tried.

To top it off, I was beginning to receive the advice that every infertile couple comes to dread, "Just relax, it will happen." After hearing it for the umpteenth time, I was ready to explode. Instead, I cried, I prayed.

I was sure God was just putting me through a test period to make me more aware of my dependence on him. After all, he just wouldn't allow me not to have children. Maybe God was simply using a little family planning of his own, and when the time was right for us, he would cause it to happen. Sometimes I was reassured by this kind of faith; many times I was not.

On one of my self-pitying days a friend called, the only one I knew who had received help for her infertility problem. In her case God had used a doctor not highly qualified in infertility treatment. She said she would not recommend him because his maternity cases always came first. But she had heard of another doctor working in a nearby teaching hospital who definitely seemed to have the qualifications of an infertility specialist. She wondered if I had heard of him. I had not. But my heart jumped with anticipation and new hope as she recited what she knew about him. After hanging up, I immediately called this newly discovered physician. Somehow, I just knew this was an answer to prayer. I was able to make an appointment for the next week.

This doctor was an infertility specialist. A doctor may become an infertility specialist by following one of two paths. Doctors who completed their formal training prior to 1973 and wanted to become knowledgeable in the infertility area had to take advantage of postgraduate training programs offered at frequent intervals in locations all around the world.

Since 1973 physicians have had the choice of obtaining their training in that same way or of going into a reproductive endocrinology fellowship. This is a formal training program of two years. When a person finishes such a program he or she may take a set of exams given by the Board of Reproductive Endocrinology and, on passing, be awarded "boards" in reproductive endocrinology. Reproductive endocrinologists take care of patients with infertility problems. They also treat patients with congenital abnormalities of their female organs, women with hormone problems, women who grow too much hair, and other related problems. Many reproductive endocrinologists also give obstetric care including delivering babies. They are trained and are qualified to give any type of obstetric and gynecologic care.

Physicians who have gained an expertise in infertility care through postgraduate studies (but not a reproductive endocrinology fellowship) can also be relied on to give expert infertility care, but in addition they often do hysterectomies, treat women for gynecologic problems, and some of them do take care of pregnant women and deliver babies. They are trained and are qualified to give any type of obstetric and gynecologic care.

If you can find a physician with either training, you can be sure that you will receive good care. The problem is that it can be hard to evaluate the competency of a physician. A reproductive endocrinologist can be more interested in research projects than in his or her patients. In addition, since there are only about 200 such individuals in the country and most of them are affiliated with medical schools, one may not be available in your community. On the other hand, a gynecologist may tell you that he or she can care for your infertility but can waste your time because he or she does not have the knowledge or expertise necessary for expert care.

It is vitally important that you get good references before you go to a physician for infertility care. Then, when you see him or her, follow the suggestions given in chapter 2. When you find a caring doctor that is an expert in infertility care, whether the training was received through a fellowship in reproductive endocrinology or through postgraduate seminars and studies is not important.

While in the waiting room that following week, I found myself overhearing the conversation of two other women who were also waiting to see the doctor. One was a woman of thirty-seven and the other looked eighteen at the most.

The younger one asked the older one if she was happy with her pregnancy. "Oh, yes," she said, "but I'll be glad when it's over. I just hope we have a boy. I've had five girls and my husband insists we have a son. He'll be furious if it's a girl."

The younger girl openly declared that she hoped she wasn't pregnant at all. "I'm too young to have a baby," she suggested matter-of-factly. "Of course, if I am pregnant, I'll get an abortion."

I couldn't believe my ears. As I hid in my magazine and

pretended not to be listening, many hard and pounding questions surfaced in my consciousness. "Why, God, why can't that woman's husband be happy with five girls? Why didn't you make me pregnant instead of this immature teenager? Then an abortion would not be necessary."

Thankfully, I was soon called in to see the doctor and my questions, for the moment, were forgotten.

After giving me a complete physical and charting my medical history, he proceeded to check my BBT. He observed that I was toward the end of my cycle, so he did an endometrial biopsy[1] and took some blood samples.

He further explained to me that he wanted my husband to bring a semen specimen so that an analysis could be performed. He encouraged me to bring my husband along on future appointments. He invited me to call if we had any questions. I would now be allowed to come on his special infertility days (meaning I would not have to sit in a waiting room with pregnant women). He also outlined some of the further tests I could expect. He estimated that in about three months, depending on whether or not any tests had to be repeated, he would complete all the necessary testing and would hopefully be able to tell us something definite.

Since I had undergone surgery for appendicitis at age eight, he had some suspicions as to what could be wrong. Previous surgery in the abdominal area can result in scar tissue and adhesions affecting the reproductive organs (something my original OB/GYN doctor would have recognized had he been more knowledgeable about infertility).

I went home thanking God he had at last found a doctor for us, a doctor who really wanted to help us have a baby. John was very eager to hear what the doctor had said. I began to tell him but soon broke down in tears. Neither he nor I understood until several years later why I spent

1. Medical terms are discussed in chapter 3 and defined in the glossary.

the next few minutes crying. My tears were partially from the frustration in being unable to find a doctor and the experience in the waiting room. But more than that, finally a doctor confirmed that we had reason for concern. For the first time we had to admit the possibility that we might never have a biological child.

2

Avoiding the Early Pitfalls

John and Sylvia

"Ve are too soon alt
und too late schmart"

This Yankee-German saying found on many kitchen
walls expresses exactly how we felt about the way we
dealt with our infertility problem in its early stages. We
were indeed too soon old and too late smart. For the fact
is that we did several things wrong initially as we dealt
with our infertility, and the mistakes we made cost us
dearly. In this chapter we want to talk about some of the
pitfalls we (and others like us) blindly, serenely, wan-
dered into. With a clearer, more informed vision, perhaps
you can avoid them.

Facing Up to the Problem

The most obvious mistake we made was our slowness
to admit that we had a problem. From many conversa-

tions with infertile couples, we know that we have not been alone in making this crucial blunder. In fact, it is by far the single most common mistake infertile couples make.

In our case it was well over two years after we tried to have a baby that we began to become serious about obtaining medical treatment. For many other couples, three, four, or even five years slip by before they are willing to face up to the problem.

Too many couples believe that their inability to achieve a pregnancy is due to something insignificant, something that given time, they can overcome by themselves. Perhaps they do not make love often enough, or perhaps too often. Maybe she is too run down and needs vitamins, or maybe they have not quite mastered the right technique of intercourse. So many couples waste precious months or even years having joyless sex or enduring frustrating abstinence all in the hope that when they do have intercourse, it will finally result in a pregnancy.

In terms of facing up to the problem of infertility, the power of denial can be enormous. To admit that one has an infertility problem seems somehow to admit to a basic human inadequacy, a humiliating failure. And who is ever ready to admit that?

Even the term *infertility* can be a stumbling block in the process of facing the problem. We have a friend who has been trying to achieve a pregnancy for at least two years but who steadfastly refuses to use the term *infertile*. "I am not infertile," she insists. Somehow in her mind infertile seems to connote sterility.[1]

When should a couple seek medical help? Thankfully, there is an easy rule of thumb for this important step. It stems from the generally accepted definition of infertility: the inability to conceive a pregnancy after a year or more

---

1. Because the word *infertility* in many minds is synonymous with sterility, some professionals are beginning to use the phrase *impaired fertility* in place of the word *infertility*.

of regular sexual relations without contraception, or the inability to carry a pregnancy to a live birth. Infertility can be *primary*, the inability to conceive or give birth, or *secondary*, the inability to have further successful pregnancies after one or more live births. If you are someone who has been trying to achieve a pregnancy for a year or more without success, or you have some reason to fear you might be infertile and you have not sought out an infertility specialist, it is important that you do so immediately.

The above rule of thumb, while generally a good guide, should not be seen, however, as sacrosanct. As Judith Stigger wisely points out:

But even a one-year "stipulated period" is arbitrary when human emotions are involved. . . . For instance, when that question arises, "Should we try one more month, or should I call a doctor?" When one prays for conception during intercourse, or when either partner begins to fear that getting pregnant might not be as automatic as had been assumed, that couple is "infertile."

Given this definition, the "stipulated period" for any couple is unique to that couple. I have a South American friend whose husband took her to a physician one month after their marriage; he was concerned because she was not yet pregnant. This is an example of a situation in which a simple explanation by a doctor relieved a couple's distress (*Coping with Infertility*, p. 18).

It is particularly important that a woman over thirty not delay seeing a physician knowledgeable in infertility evaluation and treatment if she suspects that there is an infertility problem. This is because infertility evaluation and the resulting treatments take time, and even more time is required to achieve pregnancy after the problem has been diagnosed and solved.

The Assumption of Female Infertility

Many couples assume, as we did, that the female member of the marriage is the one who has a medical problem. This assumption can be a significant stumbling block in early infertility treatment. Statistics tell us that about 30 percent of all infertility problems are due to something wrong in the female. About 30 percent are due to problems of the male. And 40 percent of all infertility cases, including ours, involve a problem in both male and female. Unless a complete infertility workup is done on both partners, the full picture of the infertility problem may not be known.

Finding the Best Medical Care

In our particular situation another mistake was also costly. When we finally reached the stage of realizing we needed a doctor, we were not selective enough about choosing one.

We went to someone who was a specialist in OB/GYN. He had a good reputation as a fine physician and a warm human being. In many respects he probably was the former, and we certainly did experience the latter, but he definitely was not the best choice for infertility evaluation and treatment.

I want to emphasize that if at your initial visit the doctor seems to approach your infertility problem in a disorganized way, chances are that you will not receive as efficient and comprehensive a workup as you need. If from the beginning the doctor does not obtain a good medical history or does not plan to test both husband and wife, or merely recommends a waiting period I suggest that you not remain with this doctor. Remember, if you have gone a year or eighteen months without becoming pregnant, you have an infertility problem and need testing right now, not "next year." Valuable time can be wasted seeing a doctor who is only mildly interested or slightly knowledgeable about treating infertility.

Dr. James T. Howard, a recognized infertility specialist, has this to say about physicians, who though they treat infertility, are not practicing state-of-the-art medical care for their infertility patients:

> We also find it disturbing that some physicians have been known to be less than assiduous in delving for the reasons behind a couple's continuing failure to conceive. One of the most common statements heard by knowledgeable specialists in the treatment of infertility from whom a second opinion is sought is, "We've had all the tests." Very often, much *too* often, that couple has *not* had "all the tests"; sometimes, even very *common*—and correctable—causes of infertility have remained undetected (*We Want to Have a Baby*, p. 3).

We and many others know from first-hand exposure what Dr. Howard is saying. A friend shared this experience with us:

Five years ago we were sent by our family practice physician to the foremost gynecologist in our area. Unknown to us at the time was that his training in infertility treatment was severely limited. He found very quickly that Bill had a low sperm count which he was convinced was our problem. The doctor said my temperature chart looked great. For the next several years he attempted to treat our infertility with artificial insemination. There were no results.

After enduring five years of expense, frustration, and the merry-go-round of hope and despair, we decided as a last resort to try Dr. Lee, a certified infertility specialist. He checked our records and asked why I had never had any exploratory surgery. I said I didn't know.

I had a laparoscopy a few weeks later with major surgery the following month. Dr. Lee did not feel Bill's sperm count was a major problem. Three months later I was pregnant.

Not all of us can be helped, but infertility specialists are now averaging a success rate of 50 percent. A couple may increase their chance for success if they consult an infertility specialist as a first resort rather than as a last. For instance, poorly done infertility surgery can cause scar tissue to form and such scar tissue can permanently reduce the chance of pregnancy below what it was before such surgery was performed.

How can you find the best medical care in your particular area? Here are some suggestions:

> Look in the Yellow Pages under gynecology and see which physicians list themselves as also doing infertility care. Some of these doctors will be capable; others will not.

Check to see which physicians in your area are listed in the Resolve *Directory of Infertility Resources*. Resolve keeps an up-to-date list of all physicians in the United States and Canada who have demonstrated interest and expertise in infertility treatment. This directory is available to Resolve members by writing Resolve, P.O. Box 474, Belmont, MA 02178.

> Most U.S. doctors interested in infertility treatment are members of the American Fertility Society, 1608 13th Ave.,S., Ste. 101, Birmingham, AL 35205.

> Young Couples International, 216 Calhoon St., Charleston, SC 29401, a newly formed organization, has a very informative newsletter and a registry of physicians who provide infertility care. The group was formed by physicians and reflects the medical perspectives on infertility.

The *Directory of Medical Specialties,* a medical reference book found in all medical libraries and most public libraries, lists all those who have completed a fellowship or have been certified in the field of reproductive endocrinology.

However, it does not include those who have obtained expertise in infertility via other training or those who have completed reproductive endocrinology training but have not yet passed their board exams.

After the initial selection of a physician, make an appointment for a consultation. This is an important step and one not to be omitted. It is possible that you will be working with this physician for a number of months or even years, and the treatment you receive at his or her hands may cost you thousands of dollars. It is essential, therefore, that you are sure you have selected the right doctor for your infertility problem before you commit yourselves to this care. When you set up such a visit, make sure it is understood that you want to talk with the doctor, and that you may or may not become a continuing patient. It is vital, we feel, for both husband and wife to attend this initial session.

Prepare for your interview. Be ready to give a complete medical history of both yourselves and your family. If possible, come with past medical records. Bring a list of questions which are important to you and do not be inhibited from using your list.

Among the questions you will want to ask are the following:

Has the physician had any additional training in infertility treatment beyond his or her residency? Hopefully you will already have obtained this information, but if not, it is important to ask.

In past years most expert infertility care was given primarily by physicians on the faculties of medical schools. However, the spread of information in the past ten years has been so dramatic that any gynecologist who desires to can become an expert in providing infertility care. Even if the doctor you consult is not practicing in a large medical center or in a medical school, he or she can give you expert help, provided the doctor has taken additional training in infertility either through postgraduate programs and seminars or through a reproductive endocrinology fellowship. The ability of infertility doctors is therefore dependent on what their interests are, on their drive to achieve excellence, and on their involvement with you the patient.

Does the physician do laparoscopies? A laparoscopy is an examination of the female organs with a special instrument passed through the abdominal wall. If a woman does not become pregnant during the process of her initial infertility evaluation, the final test is often a laparoscopy. Any doctor who does not do laparoscopies is not ultimately competent to complete a fertility examination. If a doctor is adept at microsurgery and has gained expertise in using the laser with the laparoscope, you can be even more sure he or she has expertise in infertility care.

Does the physician give priority to infertility patients? It is generally much to your advantage if the answer to the above question is "yes." More than one infertility patient has had the experience of going in for a vital test only to be told that she would have to come back next month because the doctor was at the hospital for the delivery of a baby. As one friend put it, "For us to wait another whole month was like an eternity, and it only made us more anxious."

This should almost never happen. If it does, and represents a pattern for that particular doctor, you should consider changing physicians.

If a physician does not do much infertility care, certain procedures will not be available to his or her infertility patients. For example, the washed sperm insemination technique requires a relatively expensive centrifuge. If your physician does not do washed sperm inseminations or some of the other more specialized techniques, the doctor would need to refer you to another physician for such treatment. The result is wasted time, frustration, and probably increased expense to the patient. If the doctor is interested in making infertility care a priority in his or her practice, the doctor can spend the money to obtain the instruments and invest time and effort to gain the expertise necessary to do this type of medical care. The doctor's practice can be arranged so that the infertility patient is not made to wait for the obstetric patient. It is possible to work out an arrangement with a fellow doctor whereby he or she takes care of non-infertility patients and even delivers babies for the infertility specialist during a specific time of the week so that uninterrupted care can be given to the infertility patients. The important thing is that you find a physician who is committed to giving you good and relatively uninterrupted medical care.

What are the physician's prices? A doctor should have an established price list for standard infertility tests and treatments, and he or she should not hesitate to inform you of what they are. You may also want to check whether or not the doctor is willing to accept what your insurance coverage will pay for a designated service or operation.

Assess your reactions to the physician. Were both you and your husband comfortable with the doctor and did he or she establish good rapport with you? Are you confident that the doctor has the necessary training and skills to help you? Did he or she show a genuine interest in your problem and a sensitivity to the feelings you expressed, respect your questions, and deal with them patiently? Did the doctor show evidence of "working *with* you" on the testing and treatment of your infertility rather than "working *on* you"? Some doctors do not understand the anxiety and desperation that many patients bring to their infertility treatment.

My friend Mary had already undergone a fairly exten-

sive program of tests and treatment and was getting no-
where. After the doctor gave her one more discouraging
test result, Mary burst into tears and began sharing with
the doctor her sense of depression because she was not
getting pregnant. His only response was to say, "At least
you don't die from infertility."

Infertility testing and treatment involve a tremendous
amount of emotional strain and stress under the best of
circumstances, and if your relationship with your doctor
is not a good one, it is very doubtful that you will see the
testing and treatment through to a satisfactory conclusion.

If necessary, be open to changing physicians. One should
never change physicians quickly or lightly, but on the
other hand, you should not stick with a physician through
thick and thin simply because you have already invested
a great deal of time, effort, and money in utilizing his or
her services.

When should you consider making a switch? If the following are true:

1. Your doctor is dragging out the necessary testing
(three months should be enough for most infertility testing to be completed.)

2. Your doctor does not encourage you to call him or
her with any question you have about your infertility care:
timing of tests, results of tests, etc.

3. Your doctor seems insensitive to the emotional impact of your infertility problem and this disturbs you.

4. You have prayed and have asked God to help you
honestly separate your frustration with your infertility
from your frustration with your physician, but you still
feel a deep sense of dissatisfaction with the medical treatment being received. Changing to a new doctor can cause
some guilt feelings on your part, especially if you genuinely like the physician personally. But in the long run
you may feel even more guilty if you have not given yourself the opportunity for the best medical care available.

Choosing to Delay Pregnancy

When we were married during John's last year of seminary, he was twenty-four and I was twenty-three. Since our next year or two would be filled with many adjustments and changes (including a fourteen-month missionary internship in the Philippines), it seemed wise for us to practice birth control until we became more settled. I went on "the pill." I stayed on it for approximately two years until John became the pastor of a church in New Jersey and our life became more routine. It was then time, we decided, to begin our family. By then I was twenty-five and John was twenty-six. We did not know, nor did anyone tell us, that our most fertile years were behind us.

Until recently doctors assumed that a woman's fertility level remained relatively constant until she reached forty, at which point fertility began dropping off. A new study, however, indicates that fertility drops much sooner.

More tests will have to be conducted before doctors can feel totally confident about the results, but at this point it appears that there is a possible risk in postponing pregnancy much beyond the mid-thirties.

A study, done in France and reported in a 1984 issue of the *New England Journal of Medicine*, showed that a woman's fertility rate starts dropping from the age of thirty on. Up to age thirty a woman's chance of conceiving was reported by them to be 74 percent. The study further reported that women in the thirty-one to thirty-five age group had a fertility rate of 61 percent; those beyond age thirty-five had a fertility rate of 53 percent. These percentages are somewhat low for normal marriages. The study was based on women having artificial insemination. However, the reported decreased fertility rate that comes with age is a reality.

In addition, men's sperm counts are lower now than they were in the past. Doctors have been observing a gradual decline in sperm counts during the past thirty or forty years. In the early 1800s sperm counts were normally greater than eighty to a hundred million per cc of ejaculate. Now the average male's sperm count is in the range of forty million, and we consider twenty million to be normal.

Lowered sperm count may be due to pollutants in the atmosphere, to diet, or to general lack of exercise, or to excessive exercise. It may also mean that because people are delaying their attempts to get pregnant, when they finally come to see a doctor for an infertility problem, the male's sperm count has already dropped, since age can affect sperm production.

It is interesting to note that men who have a sperm count of more than two hundred and fifty million have a higher incidence of infertility. Apparently there is something somewhat abnormal about counts that are so high.

What I am saying is that delaying your family until you are older can make it more difficult to become pregnant, not just because of the female's lessened fertility, but also because the male is somewhat less fertile.

To wait a year or two until a couple has had a chance to adjust to the marriage relationship and become somewhat established is one thing, but to wait five or six years until the couple has had a chance to take a trip to Europe, buy a boat and car, and build their dream house is something else. We feel it is important that a couple carefully consider both their age and their motives before they decide to delay having children.

In the biblical era there was a profound sense of awareness that God was in control of human lives, including one's fertility.

> Unless the LORD builds the house,
>   its builders labor in vain.
> Unless the LORD watches over the city,
>   the watchmen stand guard in vain.
> In vain you rise early
>   and stay up late,
>   toiling for food to eat—
>   for he grants sleep to those he loves.
> Sons are a heritage from the Lord,
>   children a reward from him.
> (Ps. 127:1–3)

There was a realization in that age that children were a gift from God, a gift that depended on his timetable, more than man's, his blessing more than human will and effort. Perhaps we have lost some of this humbling awareness of our dependency on God.

Ignorance Is Not Bliss

There is one more suggestion we would like to make before we end this chapter. Become informed. We were so badly lacking in basic information in the early stages of our infertility that it is almost laughable. It was not entirely our fault, of course, for in the midseventies, there was very little informative material available for the infertile couple. But in the last several years more helpful information has been published including several books and articles from a Christian perspective.

A list of materials for further reading is provided at the end of this book. But the following material is indispensable for the infertile Christian couple who want to deal with their infertility in a responsible, positive way.

The National Resolve Newsletter. Published monthly, the newsletter is a forum in which editors and readers share their insights on infertility, describe the latest infertility treatment, and provide moral support for infertile couples. To receive this newsletter you must become a member of Resolve (membership fee currently is $20.00). The membership also entitles you to other helpful information and services. The address is: RESOLVE, Inc., P.O. Box 474, Belmont, MA, 02178.

Stepping Stones. This is a free newsletter published for the infertile couple, but unlike the Resolve newsletter, it is written from a distinctively Christian point of view. It deals less with the medical side of infertility than does the National Resolve Newsletter but it does an excellent job of helping couples to cope Christianly with the tension, frustration, depression, and disappointments that infertility often entails. To obtain this valuable newsletter, write to Stepping Stones, P.O. Box 11141, Wichita, KS, 67211.

Infertility: A Guide for the Childless Couple by Barbara Eck Menning, (Englewood Cliffs, NJ: Prentice-Hall, 1977). This book is known among many infertile couples as the "bible" of infertility. It is an invaluable primer on the causes, treatment, and frustrations of infertility.

The Wedded Unmother by Kaye Halverson. (Minneapolis: Augsburg, 1981). This is a personal account of one woman's struggle with infertility. Many people find it reassuring and helpful to learn of others who have struggled with what they are experiencing. Halverson's book provides such an opportunity.

1250 Health-Care Questions Women Ask by Joe S. McIlhaney, Jr. (Grand Rapids: Baker, 1985). Written by a Christian gynecologist who has an extensive infertility practice, this book has an excellent chapter containing answers to 114 questions about infertility and illustrating many current infertility treatment procedures. The material is reliable and comprehensive but also easy to understand. It is an excellent resource for infertile couples.

These books are available at (or may be ordered through) local Christian bookstores.

3

What Constitutes a Complete Infertility Workup?

Joe S. McIlhaney, Jr., M.D.

Getting Acquainted

· A physician competent in fertility evaluation procedures will provide accurate information about the causes and treatment of infertility, dispel any misinformation you may have on the topic, have an intelligent and systematic approach to your problem, be able to project how soon you should be able to get pregnant, assuming there is a solution or treatment for your problem, and be able to counsel you about adoption options if you decide to choose that means of having a child.

Both husband and wife should be involved during the entire infertility evaluation process. Just as conceiving and raising a child should be a joint effort, so is infertility a joint concern.

The evaluation cannot take place without the husband's cooperation, since he is involved in not only the questioning and testing but possibly also in the treatment phases of the process. If both husband and wife are present at the initial interview, the couple will have a better understanding of the entire program.

Additionally, some of the procedures may require that the couple's normal sexual routine be changed. This requires the husband's support and cooperation. His attitude is much more likely to be positive and helpful if he has been involved in this effort from the start.

Finally, if the husband has met the doctor, he will feel more comfortable about calling him or her if he has any questions.

The doctor will attempt to uncover the reasons for your failure to conceive by doing a thorough evaluation of the reproductive tracts of both wife and husband. The investigation will also include obtaining a comprehensive medical history on both of you to ascertain if there is a general medical problem causing your infertility. Finally, the doctor will discuss your sexual activity to be certain that you are having proper frequency of intercourse and at the right time of the month.

During the first visit the medical history, the sexual-habits evaluation, and a complete physical examination of the wife will usually be done. If no cause is found initially, the couple is scheduled for a series of tests. Since infertility can be caused by either or both the husband and wife, it is essential that both undergo the standard tests. If, for example, the doctor finds a malfunction in the man's reproductive tract, clearing that up will not solve the couple's infertility if the woman has blocked tubes.

As stated previously, problems with the male organs cause infertility about 30 percent of the time, while female abnormalities are responsible about 30 percent of the time. A combination of factors causes about 40 percent of the problems.

The infertility evaluation can usually be completed in

two to three months, but specific problems may involve an additional few months.

Costs

The cost depends heavily on how soon your problem is diagnosed and what treatments will be necessary to eliminate it. The costs will increase as more office visits, medication, surgical procedures, and tests are required.

In calculating costs, two factors are important considerations. First, insurance policies are now beginning to cover these procedures. Second, while this care can add up to a sizable amount of money, remember that adopting a child is also quite expensive.

The following list gives the average cost for various tests and treatments for infertility in Austin, Texas, in 1986:

$100, initial office visit (consultation and examination)

$100, initial lab studies

$170, X-ray of uterus (HSG)

$60, Sims-Huhner (postcoital) test

$45, office exam each month during use of Clomid

$20, cost of the usual five Clomid pills each month

$55, cost of an ultrasound study (three or four studies can be required each month)

$80, intrauterine insemination, IUI, with washed sperm

$1,800, cost of laparoscopy (including doctor's fees, outpatient operating facility, laboratory fee)

$5,000-$6,000, cost of major surgery for scarred tubes or endometriosis

$5,000 per month, in vitro fertilization

General Advice

After obtaining your history and doing an examination, the doctor will offer you some general advice to enhance your chances of conceiving. During the first visit, for instance, I make several suggestions.

If the man wears jockey-style underwear, I advise him to switch to boxer shorts. The reason for this is that the testicles need to be cooler than the rest of the body in order to achieve optimum sperm production. Testicles normally hang outside of and away from the body for that reason. Close-fitting underwear holds them much closer to the body than does a pair of boxer shorts.

If a man's work environment or his hobbies cause prolonged heat to his genitalia (i.e., driving a truck for hours or frequent saunas), I recommend a change.

I instruct women patients to begin taking their temperatures every morning with a basal thermometer. This thermometer is necessary because it detects a narrower range of temperature than a regular fever thermometer. The thermometer should be shaken down and put at bedside every night. First thing each morning the thermometer is put under the woman's tongue for five minutes before reading and recording the results. A temperature chart should be kept faithfully for three months and brought back on subsequent visits to the doctor. This chart presents a graphic demonstration to infertility patients of the timing of their ovulation. It shows whether or not they are ovulating and helps them to schedule intercourse accordingly. Recent studies indicate that unfortunately the BBT is wrong about the exact time of ovulation in as many as 30 percent of the women who faithfully chart their temperatures. However, the BBT is still considered useful in the early stages of infertility evaluation.

The woman's basal temperature chart can also suggest to the doctor that she has a luteal phase defect (improper preparation of the lining of the uterus to receive a pregnancy). If her period starts ten days or less after ovulation, she may have an inadequate luteal phase. In either situation, the condition must be corrected before pregnancy can occur.

In 1985 an American firm began marketing an ovulation detection kit, the first nonprescription method for determining a woman's most fertile time. The kit measures a woman's LH production. When LH is detected in a woman's urine, she will ovulate during the next thirty-eight hours. Several such kits are now on the market and are very useful.

I further recommend proper frequency and timing of intercourse. No matter how fertile you are, if your sexual timing or habits are wrong you will probably be slow to achieve pregnancy. For example, I have had as patients several couples who were having intercourse only once a month, and this only at random times. Having sex about three or four times a week, spread out over the week, seems to produce the greatest chance of pregnancy. This pattern is most important to follow around ovulation time. A recent study has shown that if a woman regularly and frequently smells the odor from a man's underarm her periods will be more regular. Perhaps this is important in fertility.

I also recommend that a woman remain in bed on her back, for at least thirty minutes after each act of intercourse during the ovulation period. (She should lie on her stomach if her uterus is tipped or retroverted.) This allows the semen to pool around the cervix and facilitates the sperm's access to the uterus.

Good general health and sound lifestyle habits can have a positive effect on a person's fertility. If the woman diets excessively, is extremely obese, or exercises too strenuously, the functions of the body are changed enough to prevent normal secretion of hormones and therefore a normal menstrual cycle.

I always advise couples to avoid the following substances while they are trying to achieve pregnancy.

Cigarette smoking. Chemicals in cigarette smoke com-

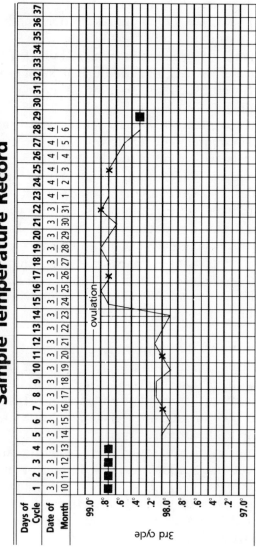

Sample Temperature Record

x—intercourse

■ menstration

Instructions:

1. Immediately after waking in the morning and before arising, eating, drinking or smoking, place the thermometer under your tongue for at least five minutes. (Do this every morning except during menstruation.)

2. Record the reading on the graph by placing a dot at the proper location (be accurate). If intercourse has taken place during the previous twenty-four hours, cross the dot (X).

3. Insert the date at top of column in space provided for date of month.

4. Consider the first day of menstrual flow as the start of a cycle. It is not essential to record the temperature during menstruation. However, indicate menstruation with a ■ on the graph starting at extreme left under number one day of cycle. As flow diminishes resume temperature recordings.

5. Any obvious reasons for temperature variation such as an infection, insomnia, or indigestion should be noted on the graph above the reading for that day.

6. If you detect ovulation by a twinge of pain low on one side of the abdomen or by a few drops of vaginal bleeding about midcycle, indicate it on the graph.

bine with red blood cells, preventing them from carrying a normal load of oxygen. If body tissues are so starved for oxygen that they cannot grow properly, it is reasonable to assume that the reproductive system may not function properly either. Studies have conclusively shown a significantly decreased fertility in male smokers and decrease fertility in female smokers.

Furthermore, once pregnancy occurs, it is imperative for the well-being of the child that the mother stop smoking. The best time to stop is before pregnancy occurs, especially if you have infertility problems.

Alcohol. Little is known about alcohol consumption and fertility. Much more is known about alcohol used during pregnancy, and none of it is good. It is my recommendation that there be no drinking or drinking only in highly controlled moderation (two to three drinks per week) for both the husband and wife who are trying to achieve pregnancy. Studies do show decreased fertility in couples when either of them drinks immoderately.

Other drugs. Even less is known about the effect of other drugs on fertility. Marijuana research shows that this drug

Steps in Infertility Workup

The tests and procedures listed below are commonly used to determine reasons for infertility and are described in detail in this chapter. A couple may not need to undergo all of them.

Female	Male
Comprehensive medical history	Comprehensive medical history
Complete physical examination	Complete physical examination
Evaluation of sex habits	Evaluation of sex habits
Examination of reproductive tract	Examination of reproductive tract
Charting of basal body temperature (checking time of ovulation and possible inadequate luteal phase)	Counseling on timing of intercourse
	Semen analysis: analysis of sperm count and health (quantity, shape, speed)
Counseling on timing of intercourse	Hormone tests
Progesterone (hormone) testing	Testicular biopsy
Endometrial biopsy	X-ray vasograph
Hysterosalpingogram	Hamster egg penetration test
Sims-Huhner (postcoital, PK) test	
Laparoscopy	

—

can affect the production of a normal egg, inhibit ovulation, and lower sperm count. People who use marijuana definitely have decreased fertility. Heroin, cocaine, barbiturates, and so on used excessively are known to cause malnutrition and therefore some degree of infertility.

The maxim concerning infertility and the use of any drug is, "Don't use the drug." If you are going to the inconvenience and expense of diagnosing your infertility and having it treated, maximize your chances for pregnancy by stopping all drugs, including cigarettes and alcohol.

Initial Tests and Evaluations for Female Infertility

A group of tests that any doctor would obtain during any thorough general checkup are also recommended for a woman with an infertility problem.

Complete blood count. This checks for anemia or a chronic blood problem that could affect both fertility and the health of the mother and the fetus.

Complete urinalysis. This checks for evidence of a chronic kidney disease, which could affect both fertility and a pregnancy.

SMA 21. This checks for any evidence of liver disease, gout, diabetes, kidney malfunction, and several other problems that can affect fertility in the female.

T3 & T4 and/or a TSH test. These check thyroid function. It is unusual for a thyroid problem to cause infertility, but it does occur and should be checked.

Rubella titer test. This tests resistance or lack of resistance to German measles (rubella) which, if contracted during pregnancy, may cause severe abnormalities in the baby. If the test shows you have no resistance to rubella, immunization should be done and for the next three months you should use good contraception. You may continue testing during this time.

TB skin test. If a woman has had tuberculosis, it may have affected the female organs and caused infertility.

Prolactin test. The prolactin level needs to be checked because this hormone can indicate a small tumor in the pituitary that could be preventing pregnancy. Not all physicians do this routinely.

Progesterone testing. Some doctors like to have a blood test for progesterone. This is done a few days after ovulation and indicates that a woman's ovary did release an egg and then developed a corpus luteum that is producing progesterone, the hormone necessary for preparing the lining of the uterus for pregnancy or causing a menstrual period to start fourteen days after ovulation if no pregnancy has occurred.

If the progesterone production is normal and the lining of the uterus is properly developed in anticipation of pregnancy, then pregnancy can occur. If the production of progesterone from the ovary is insufficient, the luteal phase is inadequate. This problem apparently stems from a lack in the corpus luteum of the cells that produce progesterone. In this situation there is nothing wrong with the lining of the uterus itself, other than the fact that it has been poorly prepared for pregnancy.

Generally a doctor will obtain one progesterone test. This will indicate at least that an ovary is capable of producing progesterone. However, the test is not conclusive in excluding the possibility of inadequate luteal phase. To use progesterone blood tests for this purpose, they must be done daily for three or four days after ovulation. Running the tests for only one month is not enough though; they must be done for several months to reach a conclusive diagnosis. This is expensive, inconvenient, and primarily a research tool. Therefore, most of the time a doctor will make the diagnosis with combined evaluation of temperature charts and an endometrial biopsy.

Endometrial biopsy. Another method of diagnosing an inadequate luteal phase is an endometrial biopsy. The lining of the uterus undergoes precise changes every day of a woman's cycle from ovulation until menstruation starts, usually on the twenty-eighth day. The lining has a corresponding precise appearance on each particular day after ovulation. If biopsy of a uterus is done on day twenty-four as determined by a temperature chart, but the tissue appears to be characteristic of day nineteen, there is an inadequate luteal phase. If the two are not within two days of each other, a luteal phase defect probably exists.

An endometrial biopsy is often done in the doctor's office, usually without anesthesia. It is a quick, but painful, procedure. An endometrial biopsy is performed by inserting into the uterus a small, hollow, round tube with a sharp lip. As it is drawn back, some of the lining of the uterus is collected. This tissue is fixed on a slide and studied under the microscope by a pathologist.

Frequently an endometrial biopsy is done at the same time as a laparoscopy (an examination which most infertile women eventually have done). I prefer this procedure since it is done with general anesthesia and causes the patient no pain. When an endometrial biopsy is done at the time of laparoscopy, the doctor will often term it a D&C. However, he or she does little dilating and only enough curetting to get a small sample of the endometrium.

A great deal of information is gained from an endometrial biopsy done after ovulation that cannot be obtained any other way.

Physical abnormalities

The following abnormalities, each of which can interfere with fertility, are evaluated during the initial physical examination.

Vaginitis. If a vaginal infection is found (trichomonas vaginitis is a likely culprit) it must be treated, as it can delay the occurrence of a pregnancy.

Growths or abnormalities in the pelvis. These may be

fibroids of the uterus, ovarian tumors, or endometriosis. Additionally, if some congenital abnormalities are found on pelvic examination these must be evaluated and may need to be treated.

Cervical stenosis. This is a narrowing of the opening into the uterus. It can prevent or make it difficult for the sperm to gain access to the uterus. This condition is often due to an earlier abortion, cervical cautery or freezing, or a cervical conization (excision of cervical tissue).

Unusually heavy or abnormal patterns of hair growth and/or moderate-to-severe acne. These symptoms can be indicative of an excess production of male hormones (even in women) and may suggest the need for hormone studies. Such studies usually, however, prove to be normal since most heavy hair growth is an inherited characteristic and not an abnormality.

Physical abnormalities. These can indicate abnormal growth patterns in the body that could be due to congenital problems such as chromosomal abnormalities. One of the most common of these is called Turner's syndrome or ovarian agenesis, a problem that requires more extensive treatment and counseling than just dealing with infertility. However, these problems occur infrequently.

Structural abnormalities. A thorough, competent infertility doctor will usually find a variety of structural abnormalities at the initial exam.

Abnormal vagina. A tough hymen can prevent proper penetration of the penis; a vaginal blockage can prevent deposition of the semen by the cervix.

Abnormal cervix. Cervical problems can inhibit fertility through abnormal cervical mucus due to cervical infection, previous cervical surgery, inadequate hormone stimulation of the cervical mucus, or a woman being allergic to her husband's sperm. Cervical stenosis (tight cervix) and mycoplasma or chlamydia cervical infections can also affect fertility.

Abnormal uterus or abnormal endometrium (uterine lining). There are many problems involving the uterus that can prevent conception, including fibroid tumors and congenital abnormalities. The inside of the uterus is called the endometrial cavity, and the lining of the inside of the uterus is called the endometrium. There may be polyps projecting from the uterine wall, fibroid tumors distorting the uterus or its cavity, or an infection of the uterus. The endometrium reflects the function of the ovaries and other hormones in the body. If these hormones are functioning abnormally, the lining of the uterus will not undergo proper changes during the female monthly cycle and will therefore not be receptive to pregnancy.

Abnormal fallopian tubes. Problems of the tubes may result from previous infection that scarred or blocked them, a previous sterilization procedure, congenital abnormalities that caused distortion of the tubes, previous tubal pregnancies, or endometriosis.

Abnormal ovaries. The ovaries may not function properly because of endometriosis, scarring from previous infection, polycystic ovarian disease, or some abnormality of hormone production by the ovary.

Abnormal hormone functioning. Since hormones control ovulation, abnormal hormone function can cause infertility. The hypothalamus, located at the base of the brain, monitors the release of hormones. This gland is the master control gland for the female cycle. Its abnormal function can cause an irregular cycle or prevent ovulation. Abnormal function of the thyroid or adrenal glands can also prevent normal ovulation.

Initial Tests and Evaluations for Male Infertility

Most gynecologists working with infertility will order only a semen analysis. If this test for sperm count and health and semen (the mucus that carries the sperm) health is normal, the husband usually needs no further testing. It is wise, therefore, that this be one of the first tests ordered for any infertile couple.

A low sperm count, unhealthy sperm, or a congenital problem are frequent problems that can cause male infertility. As stated previously, cigarette smoking can have a significant effect on sperm production. Alcohol can lead to infertility and impotence; marijuana can affect production of sperm; heroin, cocaine, and barbiturates can affect both libido (sex drive) and general health; and tranquilizers or antidepressants reduce sperm production in animals and may do the same in men.

It is important to note that sperm production that begins "today" in a man's testicles does not appear in his ejaculate for about seventy-five days. Whatever he does today, therefore, will not affect his sperm count or his sperm fertility for seventy-five days.

A urologist ordinarily treats a man with an infertility problem. I will give only a brief overview of male infertility. As previously stated, most gynecologists specializing in fertility care can order the preliminary semen tests. Further testing and treatment will require seeing a urologist.

Two things are important for a man to remember when collecting a sperm specimen for analysis.

Do not abstain from intercourse for over four or five days before collecting the specimen, because this can make the sperm count lower than it really is. Two or three days is okay, or just follow your normal frequency of intercourse.

Do not collect the specimen following withdrawal during or after intercourse. This contaminates the specimen with vaginal secretions and also makes it possible to lose part of the specimen, making it appear as though you have a lower sperm count than you do.

If the sperm analysis shows the production of few or no

sperm (a sperm count that is twenty million or higher per cc of semen is considered normal), several other tests will be performed. These include hormone tests to be sure no hormone problem exists; testicular biopsies to see if sperm can be produced; X-ray vasographies (injection of dye into the vas) to pinpoint the location of blocked sperm ducts; and testing the sperm to see if they will penetrate hamster eggs. This test gives a clue as to whether or not they can penetrate the wife's eggs. It does not produce fertilization of the hamster egg.

Treating the male usually is much simpler than treating the female, primarily because there are fewer choices for treatment and the problem can either be treated fairly easily or not at all.

An infection in the semen can be corrected, whether it is from prostatitis (inflamation of the prostate gland caused by infection), seminal vasiculitis (inflamation of the seminal vesicles), or some other type of infection. If there is a varicocele, an accumulation of veins around the testicle, the urologist may want to operate to tie off the engorged veins. The rationale behind this surgery is that the enlarged veins keep the testicle warmer than it should be. Testicles produce the best sperm counts when they are cooler than the rest of the body. When the varicocele is tied off, the testicle (or testicles) gets cooler and starts producing better sperm. Because testicular cooling may improve semen quality, you may want to apply ice to the scrotum each evening or use a THD (testicular hypothermia device ordered through your urologist or gynecologist from Repro-Med Systems, Inc., Box 191, Middletown, NY 10949) to provide cooling in a much more scientific way.

If a man does not have a varicocele but still has "bad" sperm, the doctor may try giving him Clomid or some other drug. Although the results are often unsatisfactory, their use may be worth a try.

If this does not work, intrauterine inseminations with

the husband's washed sperm can be done. Or, if that fails, in vitro fertilization or GIFT can be tried. If none of these techniques works, insemination with another man's sperm (AID) can be done.

If a man has had a vasectomy for sterilization, he can have that vasectomy reversed. A doctor who uses a micro-surgical technique can open the scrotum where the initial incision was made for the vasectomy. The scarred ends of the vas can be cut open and sewn back together so that sperm can once again flow through the reproductive tract. If the vasectomy was done recently, the husband has an excellent chance of producing normal sperm that can re-sult in a normal pregnancy. If it has been several years since the vasectomy, he has less chance of producing healthy sperm. If it has been more than ten years since a vasectomy was done, the husband may have only a 10-20 percent chance of being able to produce healthy sperm after his vas are repaired. The only way to know whether or not an operation to repair the vas will work is to try it. If the husband decides not to have this operation, or if after a vasectomy reversal inadequate sperm are pro-duced, the only alternative for pregnancy to occur is to have artificial insemination done using donor sperm.

Further Steps in Infertility Evaluation

After the couple has had the first consultation and the above-mentioned testing, the doctor will review the re-sults. Any indication of a problem should be clearly ex-plained by the doctor so that the couple will understand exactly what is going on and what will happen next.

The common causes of infertility, such as a low sperm count, are first tested. The simplest, nonsurgical tests are also done first, followed by more involved tests and treat-ments until a cause is discovered and the proper therapy found. Often the problem can be cleared up quickly and easily, and pregnancy will occur without the need to pro-ceed to the more advanced tests and procedures.

If no apparent cause for infertility was found during

the first series of questions, tests, and examinations, a hysterosalpingogram, a Sims-Huhner, and a laparoscopy test are scheduled for the woman.

Hysterosalpingogram

This X-ray test is used to view the inside of the uterus and fallopian tubes. It is a non-surgical procedure. An X-ray dye is squirted through the cervix, up into the uterus, and through the fallopian tubes so that these organs may be X-rayed and any abnormality will be outlined.

The test can show several things: whether or not the uterus is formed normally; whether or not there is scarring inside the uterus from a previous miscarriage or an operation such as an abortion; and whether or not the tubes are open. While this X-ray is not foolproof, it does give doctors a fairly reliable picture of the uterus and tubes.

Since this procedure can cause cramping, I usually have patients come in for a paracervical block on their way to the X-ray clinic. A hysterosalpingogram takes only about an hour, and is a very important part of an infertility evaluation.

Hysteroscope

When the X-ray shows abnormalities in the uterine cavity, it is usually important that they be corrected, provided they are correctable. Scarring in the uterus can cause both infertility and miscarriage, and small polyps or growths inside the uterus seemingly act like an IUD (intrauterine contraceptive device) in preventing pregnancy. Therefore it is necessary that these abnormalities be removed.

A hysteroscopy may be done in a doctor's office by using a paracervical block or in a hospital under paracervical or general anesthesia. An instrument called a hysteroscope is inserted through the cervix; it has a lens system with a fiber optic light that allows visualization of the interior of the uterus. With the hysteroscope, abnormalities inside the uterus can be seen. Small instruments are available for operations with the hysteroscope. Polyps can be removed, scars cut apart, and congenital abnormalities corrected, all without making an incision into the uterus.

Occasionally some of the abnormalities seen on the X-ray of the uterine cavity cannot be operated on with a hysteroscope. In this situation the doctor must make an incision in the abdominal wall in order to cut the uterus open from above and take out the polyps or growths.

Sims-Huhner test

While awaiting the hysterosalpingogram, or soon after, a Sims-Huhner test (SHT) can be done. This test, also called postcoital or PK, examines the cervical mucus and its reception of the husband's sperm.

The husband's ejaculate (material that comes from his penis during intercourse) is mostly mucus. Once the ejaculate is in the vagina, the sperm swim out of it and into the cervical mucus. If the cervical mucus is not receptive to the sperm, it acts as a barrier to the sperm reaching the uterine cavity.

For the SHT, several scheduling considerations are necessary. First, intercourse must take place from two to six hours prior to the scheduled office visit set up for the SHT. Second, the office visit must be scheduled one or two days before ovulation.

During the procedure the doctor will take some of the mucus from the cervix, put it on a laboratory slide, and look at it under a microscope. There should be many active sperm, and these sperm should have good direction as they swim—as though they know where they're going.

This test produces a good indication of the condition of the husband's sperm and the woman's cervical mucus as well as the interaction between the two substances. If the sperm are immobilized or killed, the mucus is "unhealthy and hostile," and the condition probably needs to be treated.

Actually, some recent studies have shown that a "good" or "bad" SHT may not be as important as previously thought. In the studies, a laparoscopy done at the right time of the month and after intercourse showed that sperm had actually traveled up into the uterus and tubes in some women with "bad" SHTs, and no sperm had reached the uterus and tubes in some women with "good" SHTs. Conclusions on this particular problem, obviously, are currently ambiguous. Nevertheless, most doctors will try to get the cervical mucus healthy and receptive to sperm, or will try to bypass unhealthy cervical mucus with the new technique called intrauterine insemination with washed sperm. (See page 111.)

It is important to understand that a Sims-Huhner test is not a substitute for a semen analysis. The SHT does not tell a great deal about the husband's overall semen specimen. To determine whether or not he is fertile, the husband must take a semen specimen to the laboratory for a competent evaluation. Just because his sperm do get into his wife's cervical mucus does not mean he is able to fertilize her. Having a Sims-Huhner test will not prevent pregnancy during the month it is performed.

Laparoscopy

When all the studies mentioned above have been done and any abnormalities have been corrected, if pregnancy still has not occurred a diagnostic laparoscopy needs to be done.

This is a minor surgical procedure that can usually be done with general anesthesia on an outpatient basis.

A laparoscopy takes about thirty minutes, unless some other procedure (laser, surgery) is done at the same time. After one is put to sleep, the physician inserts a needle through the lower edge of the navel. Three quarts of carbon dioxide gas are allowed to flow through the needle into the abdominal cavity, blowing it up like a balloon.

Either one or two incisions are made—one in the lower

edge of the navel and another just above the pubic hair-
line. Neither incision is more than a quarter of an inch
long. If only one incision is used, it is made in the lower
edge of the navel.

Through the upper incision the doctor inserts a telescope with optics so refined that the interior of the abdomen can be seen as though one were looking directly
at it. Through the lower incision the doctor inserts small
instruments such as a long probe, or an instrument with
delicate teeth to pick things up and move them around.

About half of the time the laparoscopy reveals some
abnormality in infertility patients, such as endometriosis,
adhesions, or congenital abnormalities. These abnormalities are often correctable. Occasionally, using the small
instruments that are employed during the laparoscopy,
adhesions can be cut, biopsies can be taken, and the laser
can be used without making larger incisions. At other
times the abnormalities are too major to be corrected
through these small incisions, and a major operation must
be done later.

Most doctors always arrange for a laparoscopy to be
done several days after ovulation. Occasionally a doctor
may recommend a laparoscopy before ovulation. They
normally dilate the cervix and scrape some of the uterine
lining out (D&C) at the time of the laparoscopy. The D&C
is beneficial because it gives a sample of the lining of the
uterus to send to the pathologist for evaluation. The lab
report tells whether or not this lining is responding properly to the hormones from the ovary and from other glands
in the body. This is essentially an endometrial biopsy.

Recovery from a laparoscopy takes a few days. A patient should stay in bed the evening of her surgery,
getting up only to use the bathroom. The next day she
can get up and do anything she wants, but she may not
feel like doing much.

There is some pain as a result of laparoscopy. A woman
may have shoulder pain, which is referred pain from the
diaphragm where gas bubbles are causing temporary ir-

ritation. Most of the carbon dioxide was allowed to leave the abdomen at the end of the surgery, but a small amount is always trapped inside. She may also have incision pain, but it is not excruciating and lasts only two or three days. Most women can return to full activity in two to four days, although some will be groggy and tired from the anesthesia for up to two weeks.

It is my opinion that no physician has done a complete infertility evaluation until a laparoscopy has been performed. D&C alone is not adequate, because it is the less important part of this procedure. If a doctor suggests a D&C for fertility testing, he or she is probably unfamiliar with the best techniques for the diagnosis and treatment of infertility. You should probably get a second opinion.

For example, I once had a patient whose previous physician, except for failing to do a laparoscopy, had done an adequate infertility evaluation. The X-ray of her uterus and tubes was normal. On the basis of the evaluation the woman had undergone treatment for approximately three years. Because she continued to be infertile, however, I immediately scheduled a diagnostic laparoscopy and found that both of her tubes were completely closed. The X-ray of her uterus erroneously had looked normal and the physician did not investigate further. She had wasted two or three years because her original doctor had not done a laparoscopy.

My suggestion concerning laparoscopy is this: first have all the preliminary tests done. If everything seems all right and you are under thirty years of age, wait six to twelve months to see if pregnancy will occur. If it does not, have a laparoscopy and D&C. However, if you are over thirty, or if some abnormality is detected that would be clarified by a laparoscopy, go ahead and have it done immediately.

Even though everything appears to be normal on all other exams and tests, the laparoscopy is necessary to insure that the tubes and the rest of the pelvis are normal.

Many other surgical and nonsurgical procedures can be

done to treat or diagnose a particular problem, but the foregoing material covers most of the initial studies necessary for proper evaluation of infertility.

In spite of all our modern medical knowledge and skills, after all the testing has been done, in 10 percent of the infertile couples the physician will not be able to discover the cause of their infertility. If these couples have tried unsuccessfully for four years to achieve a pregnancy, their chances for success are very poor unless they take advantage of the in vitro fertilization or GIFT procedures.

There is a more extensive discussion on the diagnosis and treatment of infertility in chapter 11 of *1250 Health-Care Questions Women Ask,* available at your local bookstore.

4

The Infertility Struggle

Sylvia

When Rachel saw that she was not bearing Jacob any children . . . she said to Jacob, 'Give me children, or I'll die!' " Gen. 30:1.

Mothers, Mothers, Everywhere

For the infertile, the pain associated with infertility can come in many shapes and from many different directions.

For me it came, for example, in the form of a comment a fourth grader in my Sunday school class made on a Mother's Day—"It's not Mother's Day for you," she said, "you're not a mom." Little did she realize the hurt her painful reminder gave me. She along with many others, didn't realize how hard it was to come to church on Mother's Day. But she was only a child and did not mean to hurt me.[1]

1. From my article in *The Banner*, May 3, 1982, p. 11.

Comments from adults can often cut the infertile couple even deeper. "What are you waiting for?" "Isn't it about time?" "Kids aren't that bad." "Just relax." "Just adopt and you'll get pregnant!" "You're trying too hard."

> One of the most popular myths concerning becoming pregnant is that "if you'll just relax and quit worrying about it, you will become pregnant." However, the *reason* you are not relaxed is that you are not getting pregnant: not the reverse! Several studies on this subject show that this type of tension does not inhibit fertility. It is normal for you to feel upset each month when you find out that you are not pregnant. This will rarely interfere with your chances of becoming pregnant.

While I was holding our four-month old niece, whose parents were visiting our church, an elder in our congregation came up to me and said, "It looks good." Smiling, he then turned to John and said, "Maybe now she'll get the idea that it is time for you to have children."

I never held another infant at church or where a group of people were present. I know this man did not mean to hurt me, but he did.

In her very moving book, *The Wedded Unmother*, Kaye Halverson describes the hurt of infertility in a way that only a person who has been there can really appreciate.

> I cried uncontrollably at almost anything: a pregnant woman walking down the street, a friend announcing her pregnancy. Baby showers became impossible for me to attend. I felt pitied, atypical, and extremely vulnerable. ... Mother's Days and holidays, formerly happy times, became difficult. Birthdays just made me feel older, without any progress toward set goals.
>
> Magazine articles were either geared at parenting or homemaking. Although I loved being a homemaker, I felt unsuccessful because we had no children. I pictured my-

self a failure, an inadequate, unfulfilled woman. I began to dislike teaching and became irritable with the children. Now I was a failure at my job, too. I lost all confidence in myself and went in and out of deep depressions. I coped publicly, but privately I fell apart (pp. 60-61).

For many couples pain can arise from hopes that are again and again dashed. Each time a period is a few days late, the infertile couple tries desperately not to get their hopes up, but inwardly they rise, only to be dashed if "George" makes his unwelcome appearance.

A poem appearing in a *Resolve* newsletter expresses so well the hopes and disappointments I so often felt.

> I am in pain.
> Someone just died.
> Who you say?
> Someone who never was.
>
> I am infertile.
> My period just came.
> I hurt so much.
>
> My own body
> Keeps reminding me
> That I am incomplete,
> I don't function properly.
>
> Why? Why? Why?
> Oh, my baby,
> Why can't you be?
> —Anonymous

Out of the Bedroom and into the Doctor's Office

One of the things many couples who are infertile soon discover is that there is a third person in their marriage—the doctor. The unseen but very real presence of their doctor is in the home of practically every infertile couple.

Even in their tenderest moments, the presence is there
lying between them and dictating the expression of their
love. Like an unwelcome conscience the presence often
whispers in their ears, "Not tonight, lovebirds, remember
ovulation occurs on Friday." On nights when neither partner feels like "making love" the presence can almost be
heard with the unspoken insistence, "Do you want to have
a baby or not?" Each month the dutiful couple is expected
to document how often and when the love act has occurred, and then is left to wonder embarrassingly, "Did
we do it often enough last month? Did we hit the right
days? Will our doctor think we don't love each other—
my goodness, a whole week with no Xs."

It is far from our intention to malign doctors. Certainly most physicians who treat infertility do so with
understanding and sensitivity. It is simply that by the
very nature of the conditions, the medical treatment for
infertility demands the doctor's involvement in the infertile couple's sex life.

Knowing that it is necessary, however, does not make
it any easier. The sexual act between a wife and husband
represents the culmination of the intimacy God intended
for married couples. Ideally, it should remain in the bedroom, but in a variety of ways, an infertile couple finds
that their sex life has been transported out of their intimate, cozy bedroom into the cold sterile confines of the
doctor's office.

The Temperature Chart

If the doctor does indeed become an unseen third party
in the marriage of the infertile, the number-one ally in
this unwelcome but necessary intrusion is the temperature chart—the infamous BBT.

I charted my basal temperature on and off for approximately seven years. I say "on and off" because, frankly, there have been times when I simply felt I needed a break from all the "hassles" and pressures involved. For me, the most irritating thing about the temperature routine was that our lovemaking often became so mechanical.

Often poorly informed doctors ask their patients to continue to take BBTs for many more months than is necessary. Some patients seem to think that continuous plotting of their temperatures will increase their chances of becoming pregnant. Usually it is sufficient for a woman to chart her BBT for three months to help confirm ovulation time if she has regular periods. If she does not have regular periods, taking temperatures is generally of no use.

A patient will need to have intercourse at the time of ovulation as indicated by BBTs and it is unnecessary to take temperatures after those first three months.

However, if a patient is taking clomiphene to regulate her ovulation, her physician will generally want her to begin taking BBTs again. Furthermore, there are specific reasons why certain patients need to take BBTs at other times.

Instead of a spontaneous act of love, having sex often became a programmed chore. It seemed more like going on duty than enjoying R and R.

John was never bothered as much about the programmed sex as I was. For him the fact that I had to take my temperature every morning became no more than a nuisance. It meant that whatever happened early in the morning was in his bailiwick and not mine since I had to remain absolutely quiet in order to obtain an accurate reading. It did become enough of a nuisance, however, for him to write a bit of doggerel about the whole temperature-taking process and the male point of view.

Ode to a Temperature Chart

Day One

Please, Sue, where are my shoes?
I'm in a hurry, no time to lose.
Are they in the closet or under the bed?
Are they by the couch or out in the shed?
Please, Sue, I'm already late,
Have to be in the office by eight.
Hey, Sue, can't you hear?
Am I not coming in very clear?

Please, Fred, don't bother me yet.
I can't help you, did you forget?
This thing in my mouth is not there for show.
I can't move as you ought to know.
Find your own shoes, dear husband, sir.
I have to take my temperature.

Day Two

Please, Sue, I love you, you know.
And this morning I just want it to show.
I've kissed you once, I've kissed you twice,
But the way you respond is akin to ice.

Please, Fred, I love you too,
But you'll just have to wait until I'm through!
See this thermometer I'm holding here?
It's really not for my health, my dear.
I love you, Fred, don't be unsure.
But first I have to take my temperature.

Day Three

Please, Sue, its Saturday morning,
And the doorbell's ringing without any warning!
I'd go myself, but wouldn't you bet,
I'm in the shower soaking wet.
Get up please, and quick as a whiz,
Put on a robe, and see who it is.
No, Fred, you get the door!

I know I sound like an awful bore,
But don't you understand my little chore?
If I've told you once, I've told you more,
Every morning before I stir,
I have to take my temperature.

Tests and Treatment

Closely tied in with the temperature chart as a source of frustration and emotional trial is the continued process of infertility testing and treatment. Many of the tests are expensive. Recently, for example, I went to the hospital for a laparoscopy. I checked into the hospital at 8 A.M. and was back home by 2 P.M. The bill was over $1,800! Thankfully, our insurance paid a percentage of the bill.

The standard operating policy of some insurance companies precludes payment for infertility testing and treatment because it is considered cosmetic in nature. The only reason our insurance company paid part of our expense was that the laparoscopy showed medical problems.

It is not only the hospital procedures which can be expensive, but routine office visits to the doctor can also be a shocker. Some infertility specialists charge a fee of $170.00 for the initial consultation visit and $40.00 or more for subsequent visits.

Medication can be almost prohibitively expensive. Some couples will need to spend hundreds of dollars a month on infertility treatment.

A fellow pastor's wife shared: "We wanted to say we tried everything medically possible to have a baby. But in doing so we are now several months behind in our medical payments. We have no money for anything else. What should we do? What does God want us to do? If we have no money for tithing, will we be blessed? Yet, if we don't try everything the doctor recommends, I'll always wonder if we did enough."

The expense might be easier to take if the results were

more certain. In our case, we did not know, and the doctor could not tell us, whether the Clomid I received would give us a baby. How long can a couple with limited income keep pumping hundreds, or even thousands, of dollars into treatment that is uncertain of success?

The only positive proof of success is pregnancy, and even then there can be crushing blows. Friends of ours who were being treated by AIH (artificial insemination with husband's sperm) had the discouragement of achieving a pregnancy twice, only to lose both babies through very early miscarriages. Finally after spending a large amount each month for medication, and enduring the ups and downs of monthly trips to the doctor for the AIH process, and then achieving two hope-soaring successes, only to be crushed with despair, this couple has called it enough, at least for now.

The timing and nature of some of the tests and treatments can also be a source of frustration and embarrassment. One of the lowest points in my whole infertility history came as a result of a PK (postcoital, Sims-Huhner) test scheduled for 9 A.M. one particular Friday morning.

At six in the morning John woke up and said, "Is it time to do our thing yet?" "No," I said, "we still have another hour to wait." "Oh, O.K.," he mumbled as he turned over, "wake me up when it's time." Ten minutes later he woke up with a start and said, "Oh, no!" "What?" I asked. "What is the matter?" He groaned, "You're not going to believe this, but I just had a 'wet dream'." He was right, I couldn't believe it! I can laugh about it now, but not then. I just broke down and cried. "How could you do this to me?" I wailed. "How am I going to tell the doctor that I can't have a PK test because my husband had a 'wet dream'?"

Holidays

"Mom's furious," Sue said. "Why?" I asked. "We're not going home for Christmas. I can't handle it. Jeff and I are going to Florida again this year. Last year was the best Christmas we'd had in several years. No tears, no self-pity, no inquisitive relatives. It just hurts too much to be at all those family gatherings."

For many couples in the midst of the infertility struggle, holidays become a burden rather than a joy. Going to Grandma's house for Christmas dinner is not something to look forward to knowing inquisitive relatives will inquire when one is going to start a family. Shopping for other people's children, hearing someone say "Christmas is for children," and knowing that sister Ellen's new baby will be the center of attention, does not make for a very merry Christmas. As Jody Earle puts it so succinctly in a Resolve Newsletter (Dec. 1984, p. 1): "At holiday time everything seems to make us hurt."

Most of you who have been traveling down the road in terms of dealing with infertility know the feelings described in this chapter. Some couples reading these lines may have only begun their infertility struggle and may be saying to themselves: "Isn't the author dramatizing things a bit too much?"

The answer, unfortunately, is "No." If anything, this chapter has only touched the surface. If you think the pathos has been overplayed, just wait.

5

Husband vs. Wife
OR
Husband and Wife?

John

The field of infertility is unique and unlike any other
medical specialty. It is the only known medical condition
that concerns more than one person. It is also the only
one where the Doctor starts out with two people and
hopes to end up with three or more![1]

Infertility is a couple's problem. It is not the problem
of an infertile wife, or an infertile husband, but an infertile
couple. Until that fact is understood, many husbands and
wives experience a great deal of additional solitary and
unnecessary pain. In many marriages in which there is
infertility, there is an excessive tendency, subtly or not so
subtly, to focus on "who is to blame" for the infertility.

1. S. A. Kaufman, *You Can Have a Baby* (New York: E. P. Dutton, 1978)
p. 9.

All too often this leads to a situation in which one partner feels superior and the other inferior; one partner feels disappointment over the other's inadequacies, and the other feels guilt for the same; one partner becomes relieved that he or she is not "at fault," the other becomes depressed, because he or she is.

For us this was a significant problem. I well remember the first time Sylvia suggested to me that I go to my doctor for a semen analysis. I nearly choked on my applesauce. "Me be checked," I exploded, "but I sent you to the doctor." It was frankly a real blow to my masculinity—and I admitted it. "But you can handle it better if there is something wrong with you," I said. "It's easier for a woman." She told me she wasn't so sure about that. By the end of the day, I had agreed to the test and I took my sample to the lab the next morning.

The following week, Sylvia went to the doctor to find out the results of a recent biopsy she had undergone, and to see if the results were back from my semen analysis. They were. Much to her surprise she learned that the problem might not be all hers. She had passed her test with flying colors but the doctor recommended that I consult a urologist and have the sperm analysis repeated. Sylvia confided in me later that it had been a load off her shoulders. She had been so sure it was her. "Ha, Ha," she had chuckled inwardly, "it might not be me after all, but you, John."

Needless to say, I was crushed. I honestly felt it was a greater blow to me because I was a male. Sylvia said, "Nonsense!" She then tried to explain how she had been feeling when she was so sure the problem had been all hers. If she couldn't give me children, she felt she was not a complete woman and would be letting me down. At times she even wondered if I was sorry I had married her.

Not only should couples resist the temptation for the husband vs. wife scenario described above, but infertile couples will do themselves a tremendous favor if they remember that each of them probably will react to infertility *per se* in a significantly different way.

In the beginning I assumed that John felt the same as I did about the fact that we could not have a baby. I was sure that he must be hurting inside as much as I was, that it bothered him when our friends had a new baby, that he deeply sympathized with me in my weary temperature charting and visits to the doctor, and that he understood when I burst into tears for no apparent reason.

In time, however, it became obvious that my assumptions were wrong. John wanted children badly and was very disappointed I did not become pregnant. But I realized that he was not hurting at the depth or with the same intensity that I was hurting. With that realization came anger. Why didn't he show more understanding for what I was going through? Why didn't he put his arms around me the first time I started crying instead of standing there with open mouth, wondering what on earth was wrong with me? Why did he give me only pat answers when I told him I was really struggling with God's will in all of this? Why did he show only lukewarm interest whenever I brought up the subject of our infertility for discussion?

The net result was increased isolation. I not only felt isolated from the people of the fertile world around me but also increasing detachment from my own husband.

SVR

Those feelings of frustration, guilt, anger, and isolation are not unusual when a couple is infertile. In many, if not most, marriages it is the woman who feels the greatest emotional involvement and who tends to suffer the most from infertility. It is, for example, typically the woman who seeks treatment first. It is the woman who initiates conversations about "their problem." It is the woman who sees the pregnant lady on every street corner. It is typically the infertile woman who reads the books and magazine articles, and for the most part, writes them too.

There are several possible reasons for this. For many women motherhood perhaps remains the number-one vocational goal, regardless of a career or job. To be a mother is something that many women see as being an essential part of their identity as a woman. A man on the other hand, though he finds identity as a father, is perhaps more apt to find identity elsewhere as well—usually in a career.

What is more, women tend to be reminded of their motherless state far more frequently than men are reminded of their fatherless state. What do women's magazines typically deal with? Homes and families. What do men's magazines deal with (the clean ones, that is)? Fishing and baseball. What do women talk about at church socials and coffee cliques? You guessed it. What do men talk about? You guessed that also.

Women get invited to the baby showers. Women will be asked by others if they are going to start their family soon. This does not mean that men cannot be devastated by infertility. Some men are.

Several years ago Sylvia wrote an article on infertility. She received several letters in response, one from a physician in Michigan who shared the profound impact infertility has had in his life:

> Having first-hand experience with infertility, we share your thoughts, feelings, reactions, and emotions and feel a very special bond to those with similar problems. For me it was a grief and loss reaction as severe as any other. It had a very real psychological effect on my whole life. It seemed like the only other people who listened, or even cared, were other infertility couples. . . . I will always be a member of the group of infertility couples, a group for whom one of life's greatest joys and deepest human emotions is but an empty void, a far-off hope.

Another individual expressed his great sorrow that he, as an only son, was not able to pass on his family name. He felt he was failing his parents.

More often, however, it is the woman who feels the greatest emotional attachment to infertility. This is a report on the findings of a survey of eighty-one infertile women and thirty-one infertile men conducted by the Department of Obstetrics and Gynecology and School of Nursing at the University of Utah:

> While over 70% of all respondents reported they had always expected to have children, more women (58%) than men (32%) felt they would miss out on a major life goal if they couldn't have children. In addition, 57% of women, but only 12% of men felt infertility was the hardest thing they had to face in life. Unfortunately, 65% of the women felt alone in dealing with infertility and 39% felt no one understood what they were going through.
>
> While women frequently reported feeling guilty (31%) or angry (49%) about their infertility, few men felt anger (10%) or guilt (0%). Similarly, more women than men reported feeling incomplete, defective, helpless or sexually inadequate. Conversely, men were more likely to separate their infertility from other aspects of their life than women.[2]

Even though these statistics suggest that in a majority of infertile marriages the wife carries the greatest emotional burden, this in no way absolves the husband from sharing the load. The Bible says, "Rejoice with those who rejoice, mourn with those who mourn" (Rom. 12:15). Unfortunately, altogether too many infertile wives mourn alone.

John is right when he emphasizes the emotional pain women feel about their infertility. In a study done in 1985, 50 percent of infertile women who responded said that

---

2. W. R. Keye, A. Deneris, T. Wilson, & J. Sullivan, Psychological Responses to Infertility; Differences Between Infertile Men and Women. Research study by the Department of Obstetrics and Gynecology and School of Nursing, University of Utah, 1981. Unpublished report.

their infertility was the greatest burden they had ever had to bear. Ten percent of the men responding said the same thing.

The intense pain many infertile women feel about their inability to conceive has made me conclude that for them having children is as basic a function as eating, breathing, and sleeping. Bearing a child seems to fulfil an essential need of a woman's body and relieves an inner craving. A man might be able to identify with this gnawing need a woman feels if it is compared to his appetite for sexual intercourse. If he were denied sex he could feel frustrated, even angry. This is not to imply that a woman must have a child or that a man must have sex to be normal; that is simply not true.

It has helped me as a man and as a physician to be aware of the vicious torment infertility inflicts on a woman and therefore I can be more sensitive as I treat her. When infertile couples understand and accept their feelings of frustration, pain, and despair as being valid, they can deal more positively with them.

As a minister I would like to be able to say that I was quick to gain the understanding that infertility for Sylvia was a much greater disappointment than it was for me. But I cannot say that. I was slow, shamefully slow, in coming to the realization that her hurts, frustration, and pain were strong and deep. The truth is that it was not until well into our infertility experience that I began to truly empathize with what Sylvia was feeling. There was no magic moment when this happened, no sudden breakthrough in which it all came together. Rather it was a long series of insights and incidents which together brought me to the point of being able to say to Sylvia, "I think I understand what you were going through."

There was, however, one experience that began the process:

I was making a hospital visit to a parishioner who had

undergone a laparatomy to correct some damage to her fallopian tubes. She tried to sound cheerful, but she was in fact depressed.

She shared with me that her husband had really not wanted her to have this surgery. "Frankly," she said, "he doesn't even care if we have a baby or not." She also confided in me that, when she had told him she wanted to try everything she could to have a child, he had just shrugged his shoulders and said, "Surgery is expensive, you know. You have already had one operation, how many more times do we have to go through this?"

As I left the hospital, I was angry. I was ready to drive over to this woman's husband, grab him by the shirt collar, and say, "You insensitive clod! Don't you realize how much your wife is hurting? Don't you know she needs your support and understanding?"

But before I had half-practiced my little "sermon," some questions began to creep slowly, but resolutely, into my consciousness. "Was I any better? How much understanding did I show my wife? How much support did she really receive from me?" The light was beginning to dawn.

In all honesty, it was not until we began thinking of writing this book, and I started to do the reading and research that such a book required, that I began to fully recognize how superficial my understanding of Sylvia's pain had been. Truly, I had tried to heal her wounds lightly (Jer. 6:14). I know there are many husbands who have been just as insensitive as I was.

6

Beginning to Cope with Infertility

John and Sylvia

While there are no simple solutions for dealing with the frustrations and pain outlined in the previous two chapters, one does not simply have to sit back and passively suffer. There are some things that one can do to begin coping with infertility.

Needed: A Temporary Reprieve

Take a break occasionally. It may be healthy on rare occasions to simply take a short respite from medical treatment if such treatment really begins to become emotionally draining. This should never be done wantonly or without consulting your physician, but your overall well-being may necessitate temporary breaks of a month or more from your BBT charting and treatment routine.

Be honest about it! Don't lie to yourself or your doctor. Many infertile couples, for example, have a tendency to cheat on their temperature chart. They become tired of

programmed sex, and they let a month go by without
making any conscious effort to hit the "right days." At the
end of the month, the chart looks like a barren wasteland
in the region where X's should be sprouting. Instead of
facing up to and being honest with the doctor about not
having intercourse on those days, couples fudge the record
by pencilling in a few X's. This is a cover-up, plain and
simple, but many couples practice it at one time or
another.

Sometimes I would purposely not make love with John
on my most fertile days. Strange as it may seem, I wanted
to have a ready excuse at the end of the month for the
fact that I did not become pregnant.

I wanted to be able to say to myself, "Why of course,
Sylvia, you didn't become pregnant. You didn't make love
on the right day. Next month if you have intercourse on
the key days you'll get pregnant." This was my defense
mechanism for handling my monthly depression when
my period came.

I needed this defense, but at the same time I felt guilty
and angry. I could never shake the gnawing realization
that I had let another month slip by without doing all I
could to conceive a baby. I also could not escape the fact
that I was wasting precious dollars which we could ill
afford.

Following such a month I felt very uneasy thinking
about my upcoming doctor's appointment. Should I skip
my appointment? Would it be better to leave my chart at
home? Should I lie? Would he look at my chart and ask
why we didn't have intercourse the days he recom -
mended?

Instead of this kind of deceptive and self-defeating be-
havior, tell the doctor exactly how you feel. If you haven't
followed the recommended interval for intercourse during
the key days, tell your doctor that and why. If you are at
the point where you do not want to record the tempera-

ture for awhile, say so. Chances are that your doctor will understand.

Strengthen Marital Relationships

Communicate, Communicate, Communicate! The act of communication between husband and wife is vitally important if the stresses and strains that accompany infertility are to be dealt with most effectively.

Bill and Jan were married shortly after high school. On their farm they worked side-by-side, day-in and day-out, and they became extremely close as husband and wife. There were several family crises in which they were able to be most helpful to each other. There were few things they did not talk about together, including their infertility.

In time they considered adopting a child. But much to their chagrin the social worker informed Bill and Jan that the agency required adoptive couples to use birth control for a few months prior to, and one year following, the placement of a baby in their home.

Bill said, "We have never used birth control and we are not going to begin doing so now. If that is the requirement, adoption is out for us." Jan agreed.

From that time on Bill and Jan rarely shared their disappointment in being unable to have children.

A few years later Jan had a nervous breakdown. At first no one understood why. Finally a wise infertile friend helped Bill and Jan to realize that each was hurting because they had no child, but each had been hurting alone.

All too often husbands and wives do not talk together about the frustrations they feel. There may be many reasons for this. It is possible, as described in the last chapter, that one partner does not feel as much emotional involvement with the infertility problem as the other partner, or one partner may be feeling a lot of guilt because he or she perceives himself or herself as "the problem." Possibly the lack of communication with respect to infertility is indicative of the general lack of communication in the marriage.

Whatever the reason for lack of communication, infertility is such an anxiety-producing experience that couples need to talk about it together. Even if one partner is handling infertility well and has no need to share frustrations, he or she may have to be willing to patiently and lovingly listen to the other partner's needs.

Having said this, however, it must be added that one partner may be inclined to dwell on the infertility problem and let it dominate the relationship. This can be equally destructive. To avoid that problem, some couples exercise what they call "The Twenty-Minute Rule." Having discussed their infertility often and in depth in the past, they have agreed that if one of them brings up a topic related to their infertility, they will discuss it for twenty minutes and no longer, before they move on to another subject. We think this is a good rule.

Merle Bomardierie puts it so well when she suggests:

> When this technique is applied, she talks less about infertility. She crystallizes her message because it has to be quick or she'll miss her chance. He listens intently because he knows he doesn't have to listen all night. She feels better because she's no longer driving him crazy and because, finally, she feels listened to. He feels better because he doesn't have to listen so long and because he can tell that now she really feels listened to. And best of all, they have the rest of the evening to talk about or do something else.
>
> Less is more in this instance (National Resolve Newsletter, Dec., 1983, p. 5).

Practice the art of sensitive caring. Be aware of where the other partner is emotionally and what you can do to help meet his or her needs.

For a husband, this may include doing something special for your wife during that special time of the month when you are both waiting to see whether or not her period will come. Tension can run high during such a time and a nice dinner out, an unexpected gift, or a special effort at tenderness can help relieve the anxiety. For the wife, sensitivity may include working to build up his self-confidence and giving him assurance that it is not the ability to father a child that makes someone a man. This is all part of what real love is in marriage, a love which should be patterned after 1 Cor. 13:4–7:

> Love is patient, love is kind. It does not envy, it does not boast, it is not proud. It is not rude, it is not self-seeking, it is not easily angered, it keeps no record of wrongs. Love does not delight in evil but rejoices with the truth. It always protects, always trusts, always hopes, always perseveres. (Living Bible)

Involve both partners. It is very important that both husband and wife become involved as much as possible in the infertility testing and treatment. We strongly recommend that both husband and wife go to the initial appointment with the doctor and to all subsequent appointments as well (where this is feasible). This will help to build the mutual support and understanding that is so necessary if the infertility problem is to be faced together.

It is also recommended that husbands help their wives as much as possible with the hateful chore of charting the BBT. We know of one couple's decision to let the husband do all the actual charting. He doesn't even let his wife see the chart until the month is over. This relieves her from the anxiety of wondering where she is in her cycle and becoming alternately excited and depressed as she sees the dips and valleys her BBT may bring.

Reach Out to Others

Nourish relationships with those who understand. Find other couples or individuals who have an infertility problem and with whom you can share mutual concerns. The most pressing need for finding someone to genuinely relate to in terms of the infertility struggle may be experienced by the woman. According to Dr. Anthony Labrum of the Department of OB/GYN and Psychiatry at the University of Rochester School of Medicine, "Probably the most important thing for people who have problems with various aspects of reproduction is that they not feel isolated. They need to feel open and free to talk about their problems without a sense of fear that what they say may be uncomfortable for the people listening to them" (Asprooth, National Resolve Newsletter, June 1982, p. 4).

This is one of the areas in which Resolve can really help. One of the primary functions of the local chapters of this organization is to establish infertility support groups. These groups generally consist of four to eight infertile couples who are willing to learn from and support each other.

While sitting in a doctor's office in 1977 I first read about Resolve in a national magazine. I wrote for information. The first newsletter did wonders. It told me my feelings were normal, that I was "Okay." I discovered that there were many other couples whose friends told them to relax, that other women felt as if everyone else was pregnant, that other wives too felt isolated from husbands and seemingly insensitive families and friends.

When we moved to Sioux Falls, I met two other infertile women through contacts with Resolve. We talked often. Eventually we formed a twelve-week support group. For me that was one of the most helpful things I did in coming to grips with my own feelings.

If there is a Resolve chapter in your community, ask them if there is a support group you can join. If there is no Resolve chapter, maybe you should think of starting one. Contact the Resolve headquarters in Belmont, Mass., P.O. Box 474, 02178, telephone 617-484-2424. At the very least, find one or more couples who have an infertility problem and develop a close friendship with them. If you are a Christian, you will want to find one or more Christian couples with whom you can share not only the emotional upheavals of infertility but the spiritual and ethical struggles as well. Since one of six couples has an infertility problem, there are undoubtedly couples within your church family who are experiencing some of the same struggles you are. To have an infertility problem and not be able to share your frustrations and feelings with others who understand can add to the desolation.

Develop a sense of humor. Infertility is no joke. Everyone who has been there knows that full well. But many couples become so intense, so obsessed with their infertility, that they can no longer laugh at anything, least of all their infertility.

It has been our experience that there has been healing when we have been able to sit back and laugh at some of the ludicrous experiences we or others have had. We still chuckle over an experience a friend of ours related to us:

When I was ushered into the urologist's office, he handed me a container (six ounces or more), pointed me in the direction of the lavatory, and said, "Will you go in there please, and give me a specimen—you don't have to fill it." "Fill it?" I thought to myself. "Who does he think I am anyway?" It took me a few minutes but I finally managed to "psych" myself up for what had to be done. I was just busily concentrating on the duty at hand when the doctor knocked on the door and asked, "Are you finished yet?" "No, doctor," I shouted, "this is going to take me awhile to do!" "Oh, no," he said, "What kind of specimen are you giving me?" "Semen," I replied. There was silence on the other side of the door. Finally he blurted, "But I wanted a urine specimen."

On another occasion, the same friend was, in fact, asked to go to the public lavatory and provide a semen specimen. He was in the very act when the toilet next to him started to overflow.

This friend is now able to laugh over his experiences, humiliating as they were at the time. That kind of laughter is healthy for the infertile person and helps relieve some of the tension and bitterness that infertility can bring.

Mobilize Your Emotions

Learn to control the holidays rather than letting them control you. How does the childless couple remain joyful during these joyous times of the year?

Here are a few helpful suggestions adapted from the *Portland Area Resolve Newsletter* (Nov. 1980):

1. Recognize and accept your feelings of loss and grief over what might have been. These are legitimate emotions, but try not to dwell on them. Avoid situations that are especially painful. Know your limitations.
2. Do something for someone else less fortunate. Make small gifts to charities, nursing homes, children's organizations. Keep busy. Bake for someone who can't. Visit a friend.
3. Recognize the holiday for what it is in itself, not how it affects you. Learn to concentrate on the real meaning of Christmas, Thanksgiving, and Easter, not on the commercial and social trimmings that accompany these events.
4. Share your feelings and emotions with your spouse. Work at keeping the two of you a family with your own traditions and celebrations.
5. Do something special to help you feel good about yourself during the holiday season. Treat yourself to a new hairstyle. Buy a new dress. Give yourself time to read a good book. If finances permit, take a holiday vacation.
6. As the new year approaches, set goals for yourself. Look to the future. See a new perspective and re-

member what you have already been through together with the help of the Lord.

Practice personal prayer. We will talk more about prayer and infertility in a later chapter, but for now we simply want to say this. If you have allowed the frustrations, the pain, and the difficult decisions that accompany infertility to wear you down and to gnaw away at your emotional reserves while you have not consistently been taking these concerns to the Lord, you are not plugged in to the "power" you need to cope effectively. Evelyn Christiansen, the author of the best-selling book, *What Happens When Women Pray*, puts it beautifully when she says:

> One day my husband [the pastor] walked out of the sanctuary of our church and encountered our custodian fairly dripping with perspiration. He was a giant of a Christian, but was gradually losing his ability to think and work effectively because of hardening of the arteries. As my husband saw him struggling with the vacuum cleaner, he looked down, and there lying on the floor was the plug. The dear man had vacuumed the whole auditorium and didn't have the plug in the outlet!
>
> Isn't that what happens to many of us! We work, we pull, we struggle, and we plan until we're utterly exhausted, but we have forgotten to plug into the source of power. And that source of power is prayer . . . (p. 18).

7

Friends, Family, and Fellow Christians

John and Sylvia

Dr. James Dobson, well known for his "Focus on the Family" radio program, devoted a broadcast (May 4, 1982) to the infertile Christian couple. In that program he related an experience that gets at the heart of this chapter. The incident deals with the reactions of friends who found it difficult to accept the fact that he and his wife, Shirley, had decided to postpone having children until he was through with his postgraduate education. As Dr. Dobson puts it:

> And I'll never forget what happened. It was in the fourth or fifth year of our marriage, and we had a lot of friends over to our house, the people we love most and those that love us. All night long the topic of conversation was "When are Jim and Shirley going to have a baby." It began to get monotonous. It began to get more and more insulting. And then it began to have sexual innuendos. At one point,

we were all in the living room and one person who was
there said something that was really crude, really rude.
And I don't remember what I said, but I had had enough.
And man, I mean to tell you, I leveled everybody in that
room. I said something to the effect that, "Hey, wait a
minute, I've got a message for you guys. I want you to
open your ears and hear it. Because I don't know if you
care about my friendship. But if you do, you will shut up
about this subject and you will never mention it again,
because it is nobody's business but Shirley's and mine. If
we do decide to have a child, you will definitely know
before the delivery. But until then I want you to keep
your nose out of our business!"

The living room just suddenly became empty. People
disappeared in all directions. I found myself standing in
the room by myself. But it was the last time anybody
mentioned that subject.

This incident points up the fact that infertility does not
only put a strain on one's own emotional well-being, and
one's marriage, but it can also put a tremendous strain on
one's relationships with others. Therefore, this chapter is
devoted to the following questions: How does an infertile
couple deal with well-meaning but sometimes insensitive
friends, family members, and fellow Christians? What do
we tell them about our infertility? How do we tell them?
What do we do if they hurt us?

What Do You Say to a Friendly Lady?

Before we talk about how we should relate to friends,
family members, and fellow Christians, perhaps we should
go a step beyond that and talk about how we should deal
with people who are relative strangers. For example, what
do you say to a lady you meet at the laundromat while
you are both drying your clothes, or the cheerful grandma
sitting next to you on the airplane? You know the scenario.

You begin a casual conversation. She asks you if you are employed and you ask her in return. Almost inevitably the question is raised by the other party, "How many children do you have?" For most people this question is no more threatening than asking them if they would like a piece of gum, but a person who is childless may find such a question tough to handle. On the one hand, to say simply that you don't have any children often leaves the other person thinking, "So she is one of *those* kind—the liberated woman who wants a career but no kids. I'm glad I'm not like that." Even if the other person is not thinking that (and most often she probably is not) you assume she is.

On the other hand, it is certainly unnecessary to explain your childless state to this other person, someone you have never met before and probably will never meet again. Dr. Dobson, in the program we mentioned earlier, suggests rather emphatically that we do not owe anyone an explanation. He suggests, "The decision to have children or the reason why you can't are nobody's business. That belongs only to the husband and wife. They're under obligation to no one to divulge that information."

While agreeing with Dr. Dobson that the infertile couple does not owe a stranger an explanation, we feel in the above scenario, that to simply say, "We have no children" is not quite adequate. We would suggest that a couple who is actively trying to have a child but is not yet successful, say something like, "None yet, but we're still hoping." Couples who are beyond the point of bearing children can say something like, "No, unfortunately, we were never blessed with any." A short, brief response like the above does two things: It answers the question they have asked effectively. It also avoids wrong assumptions.

Usually this kind of response will be enough for

strangers and casual acquaintances and they will not pursue the matter further. If they should be so impolite as to do so, simply tell them tactfully and sensitively, but clearly, that you would rather not talk about it.

What Do You Say to Aunt Tess?

By far the greater problem, as intimated at the beginning of this chapter, is learning how to handle the attitudes and remarks of people close to us, good friends and members of the family. This is a difficult area to discuss because beyond a doubt, most infertile couples have friends and family members who would never intentionally hurt them. And yet, in spite of not meaning to, friends and family members can add to the infertile couple's burden. Such seemingly innocent things as trying to cheer the childless couple by telling them "how lucky they are," or calling them with ecstatic excitement every time someone in the family or circle of friends has a newborn, can add salt to the wound, even though the one doing it has absolutely no idea he or she has a salt shaker in hand. Add to this the usual problem of infertile couples being invited to parties and family gatherings where children are one of the primary topics of conversation, and it becomes evident that friends and family can become unwitting contributors to the infertile couple's often growing sense of resentment and hurt.

There are at least several things an infertile couple can do to help lessen the hurt that friends and family members sometimes bring into their lives.

Some openness is recommended

Not wanting to be open with strangers and casual acquaintances about your longing to have a baby is one thing, but keeping friends and family members completely in the dark is quite another.

Many infertile couples, however, do keep those close

friends and family members very much in the dark. It is an embarrassment for them to have others know they have a problem. They feel somehow guilty about it, as if they personally were responsible for the fact that their bodies are not working properly. For one reason or another, infertility is perceived as something which at all costs must never be discussed.

This is borne out by the fact that many of those who have become more open about their infertility, speak of it as "coming out of the closet." Barbara Eck Menning, the founder of Resolve, wrote an insightful article on this very subject (National Resolve Newsletter, Feb., 1978, p. 1). She said:

> I'd like to have a nickel for every time a person has said or written, "It feels so good to come out of the closet at last!" In my 5 years of infertility counseling, my reaction has always been the same. What were you doing in there in the first place? WHO put you in the closet? Society? Family and friends? Or did you go in there all by yourself?!
>
> A recent story on infertility in a popular magazine begins: "When Lisa and Steve Anderson married..." A glance at the footnote reassures us that this is not their REAL name. "Why not?" I asked myself. "Are they having donor insemination? Have they done something wrong?" Reading on I find that the "Andersons" are only guilty of being infertile.
>
> When a story or media piece about infertility appears with anonymous characters or pseudonyms we continue to feed the age-old myth that infertility carries a stigma— that we are either guilty of something, or at the very least, pitiful. Neither is true!

Right on, Barbara! It is true, of course, that some couples who keep their infertility a secret do so because they believe they have a very good chance of eventually attaining a pregnancy and childbirth and they reason that it is foolish to tell other people about their problem if they will shortly overcome it. This sounds reasonable, but is it?

Of all those who seek medical treatment for infertility, only about 50 percent will eventually achieve pregnancy and childbirth. And many of those who do finally achieve success only do so after years of treatment. Therefore, keeping your problem a secret from others, especially those close to you, on the basis of the "iffy" belief that you will soon achieve a pregnancy and birth is fallacious at best.

It is our conviction that many infertile couples have endured unnecessary hurt simply because they have not told close friends and family members that they are facing an infertility problem. Once a couple shares with parents, siblings, friends, and possibly fellow workers, that they are trying to have a baby and are getting medical help, it is amazing how the silly questions disappear, the once seemingly funny jokes are never said, and the supposedly friendly jibes are never again launched. In our dealing with infertility, we have always tried to be open with friends and especially with family, and in return we have seldom experienced the kind of hurt that so many have, who for some reason, have kept their infertility a secret sorrow.

An infertile acquaintance shared this experience:

It was at the annual family Christmas gathering that my sister-in-law, Jane, shared the unexpected news that she was pregnant. It was difficult for me to hear, but after ten years of experiencing infertility in my life, I had learned to live with such "joyful" news. Shortly after the announcement I worked up the courage to walk over to Jane, and I asked if she and Mike (her husband) had chosen names already.

"No," she answered, "It's still a bit early, and we're in a state of shock."

"Well," I suggested lightly, "Why don't you use the names we have picked out, it looks as if we won't need them." And then for the first time I shared my infertility experience with Jane. She was shocked. Mike's mom had repeatedly assured her that I was into dogs, not kids.

On the other hand, we are not suggesting that a couple has to lay out all the intimate details of their infertility problem and treatment before every close friend and relative. Some selectivity is advised. Couples, for example, who are considering AID or in vitro fertilization (the "test-tube" baby technique) may not want to divulge that information because they may run the risk of a judgmental and uninformed, negative response. Some infertile couples also have friends or relatives who are prone to gossip, the giving of pat answers, or as Dobson puts it to become "really crude, really rude." Obviously the amount of openness the infertile couple will want to extend to such persons will be extremely limited. The couple may even be forced to adopt Dobson's blunt approach and tell such people, when they curiously and persistently inquire into the subject, that it is not up for discussion, period.

In general the amount of openness depends on the trust level that you have established with those close to you. If they are people who you can really trust, who do in fact have your very best interest at heart, and who will listen to you without trying to put you down, a certain amount of openness with them about your condition will be very helpful.

Patiently and kindly correct mistakenly held ideas

One mother sent the following in a letter to her married son who was experiencing infertility in his marriage:

> Your father read a bit of Dear Abby which indicated that too-tight underpants and pants could make sperm inactive. He was going to cut that out and send it to you— possibly with the suggestion that you switch to boxer shorts or something. I didn't know if you wore your clothes that tight or not" (*The Washington, D.C. Resolve Newsletter*, May 1981, p. 3).

We don't know how this man reacted to such a letter from his mother, but it could very easily have exasperated him. It is easy to imagine him saying to himself, "How dumb does my mom think I am? I've been wearing boxer shorts for the last four years and she comes along and thinks she's telling me something brand new. I just don't believe it."

We can imagine that many of us might react in a similar vein when a dear aunt tries to "cheer you up" by telling you about her sister's niece who was infertile for eight years and now has four kids; or when your mother-in-law tells you of at least six couples who adopted and within the year had a baby "of their own"; or when a dear friend cheerfully suggests that you are "too uptight" and that what you need to do is "simply relax," or "take a second honeymoon."

We do not believe, however, that exasperation—or its first cousin, anger—is either very helpful or very Christian in dealing with this kind of situation. The people mean well. They are honestly trying to help. Their motive invariably is love. Their major fault is ignorance.

The Christian approach, then, is to help remove their ignorance by kindly and tactfully informing them of the facts. The son who received the boxer shorts "news flash" probably needs to do no more than tell his mom, "Thanks, Mom, but I'm already wearing them and on the advice of my doctor I've been doing that for four years now." The infertile couple who is told that adoption often brings a pregnancy ought to politely inform the advisor that adoptive parents later become biological parents only 5 percent of the time. And that dear person who tells the infertile friends to "relax and it will happen" must simply be told that there is a medical reason in 90 percent of all infertility cases and no amount of relaxation will help until the medical problem is solved.

*Remember that those close to you may be hurting in
their own way over your infertility*

This is an important thing to remember, especially in
dealing with your parents. You may be grieving over the
fact that you have no child, but they may be grieving over
the fact that they have no grandchild to cherish from your
marriage. Infertility may be threatening to dash your
hopes, but it may also be threatening to dash theirs.

What is more, many parents often carry a certain
amount of guilt over their children's infertility. The following incident involving people whom we will call Jennie and Joe makes the point clearly.

Joe's parents knew all about our infertility problems.
We had kept them informed on what was wrong and which
doctor we were seeing. We must have told them a dozen
times that I was perfectly healthy (as far as the doctor
could tell) but that Joe had an extremely low sperm count
and poor motility. We had also told them that the doctor
speculated that the problems might have resulted from a
childhood bicycle accident in which Joe's scrotum had
been injured and an infection had set in.

Even though we had told Joe's parents over and over
again what the main problem seemed to be, every time
we talked to them about our infertility, Joe's mother would
ask, "Didn't they find anything wrong with Jennie?" After
about the fourth time in a year that this question popped
up, Joe and I became very irritated. Thankfully, we tried
not to let it show. One night after talking about the attitude of Joe's mother, both of us came to the same conclusion at the same time. Joe's mother felt guilty. She blamed
herself for Joe's near sterility. When it became apparent
that we were probably not going to have a baby, Joe's
mother had probably said to herself a hundred times: "If
only I had been careful about where Joe rode his bike" or
"If only we had gotten better medical treatment when Joe

injured himself." After thinking this all through, Joe and I concluded that his parents probably hoped in a way that there was something wrong with me because then they would not feel solely responsible for our infertility. This helped us to deal with Joe's parents with much more understanding.

All of us need to have that kind of understanding in dealing with those who love us. Until we do, we will be prone to react with irritation instead of compassion.

What Do You Say to Rev. Goodman?

Unfortunately, the church can also become an unwitting culprit in adding to the infertile couple's hurt. A friend of ours related, for example, that she once left a Mother's Day service in tears because the minister had emphasized the joys of being a mother and criticized in no uncertain terms the increasing number of women who wanted a career and who were selfishly deciding not to have children. Our friend asked in exasperation, "Doesn't he realize that some of us would love to have children, but cannot? He always lumps all the childless in the same boat. Doesn't he realize I have my career because it means that at least in that area of my life, I can be successful?"

The church can hurt the infertile couple simply because it is generally so family-oriented. In many churches, especially in recent years, children have come to play prominent roles in the life of the church. In many congregations, children come to the front of the sanctuary each Sunday for a children's sermon. They also present a yearly Christmas program, and Sunday school classes often provide special music. Many infertile people cannot help but wonder, sometimes almost despairingly, as they watch cute toddlers walking up to the front of church to sing or participate in the worship service, "Will my little boy or girl ever be among them?"

In many churches the women's groups also seem particularly structured for mothers. In several of the Bible discussion groups that Sylvia has been in, the lessons have centered on topics such as "Women in the Bible" or "The Christian Marriage." Usually such discussions have revolved a great deal around children. If the Bible study itself did not, the social time following the Bible study inevitably did.

After you have frankly told friends and family members about your infertility problem, you may find it very helpful to exercise a certain amount of openness to your fellow believers in your congregation. Again, we are not suggesting a public announcement in the church bulletin saying, "Mr. and Mrs. John Jones want to inform you that they are infertile." But if helping in the nursery really becomes painful to you, decline this avenue of service for a time and honestly tell the person in charge why. If your minister has preached the type of sermon mentioned above, be kind enough to tell him of your reaction. He undoubtedly had no idea he hurt you and you can be 99 percent certain he will never be insensitive to the infertile couples in his congregation again. If you're going to the hospital for surgery to help correct your infertility problem, be willing to ask for prayer during the prayer and share time of your church. The Bible tells us to "carry each other's burdens" (Gal. 6:2), but how can others help us do that if they do not know what our burdens are?

8

Infertility and the Christian Faith

John

The Christian infertile couple faces some unique questions and challenges which will not confront their non-Christian counterparts.

The Great Question

For many couples there is one question which gets at the heart of their spiritual struggle with infertility: "Dear God, why can't we have a baby? You know how desperately we want a child. You understand how difficult it is for us when friends all around have started their families and ask us why we don't start ours. You have seen our tears. You have heard our prayers. Why then have you allowed us to suffer this way? Why haven't you granted us the laughter of little children? Why? Why? Why?"

The question "Why" is certainly not new (the Book of Job raised the same question long ago), nor is it a question limited to the infertile. It is a question asked by many of

God's children at one time or another in their lives. It is
the question asked by parents who lose their four-year-
old daughter to leukemia while the child's ninety-year-old
grandfather lives on in good health. It is asked by the
twenty-three-year-old seminary graduate who is diagnosed as having an incurable brain tumor a week before
leaving for missionary duty in the Philippines. It is the
question raised by the thirty-year-old single school teacher
who has not found a life partner though she so desperately
wants one.

Knowing that the question is not unique for the infertile, however, does not make the question any less real or
intense. "Why" cries out for an answer.

In trying to come to terms with this question, we need
to recognize that traditionally three main possibilities have
surfaced for suffering in our lives. They are: to show the
results of sin, to strengthen the believer, and to glorify
God.

To show the results of sin

In discussing this as a possible reason for suffering infertility I want to be extremely careful. For I know that
many couples struggle deeply with the question of guilt
as it relates to their infertility. They ask, "Why is God
punishing us this way? Is it because we were intimate
before we were married? Is it because I masturbated when
I was younger? Could it be the result of his anger over the
brief affair I had with my secretary six years ago?"

Well, what about it? Could our infertility be a result of
sin in our lives? There are many writers in the infertility
field (including Christians) who tend to "pooh-pooh" this
possibility. They suggest that because God is a God of
love, he would never punish sin with such an awful scourge
as infertility.

I would like to respectfully and carefully disagree. When
someone, for example, engages in a promiscuous lifestyle
and contracts venereal disease which in turn leaves such

scarring in the reproductive organs that infertility results, is that not sin related? God can and does punish sins. There is ample biblical evidence of that. The Bible also contains evidence that God did, on occasion, punish sins with infertility.

Abimelech in the days of Abraham is a case in point. Abimelech earned God's displeasure by taking Sarah as his wife. He had done this innocently, of course, because Abraham had told Abimelech she was his sister. Because of Abimelech's ignorance, God revealed to him in a dream that Sarah was Abraham's wife and Abimelech was warned to return her. Then, "Abraham prayed to God, and God healed Abimelech, his wife and his slave girls so they could have children again, for the Lord had closed up every womb in Abimelech's household because of Abraham's wife, Sarah" (Gen. 20:17–18).

Possibly Michal, wife of David, was infertile because of her sin. She mocked David when David danced before the Lord celebrating the return of the Ark after its captivity by the Philistines. The closing verse of 2 Samuel 6 informs us with somber emphasis: "And Michal daughter of Saul had no children to the day of her death."

There are two reasons, however, why we should be extremely careful before identifying infertility as the result of sin in our lives. In the first place, the Bible contains many warnings against the quick and unjustified identification of suffering with sin. In the Old Testament the three friends of Job—Elihu, Eliphaz, and Bildad—tried to convince Job that the reason he was suffering so much was because of some sin in his life, but they were wrong. Philip Yancey in his very lucid and perceptive book, *Where Is God When It Hurts,* correctly points out:

> Nobody deserved suffering less than Job, and yet few have suffered more. Sometimes God does send suffering as punishment (as in the ten plagues of Egypt), *but you cannot argue backwards,* as Job's friends tried to do, and

assume that each incident of suffering can be linked to a specific failure. God Himself contradicted their accusations (p. 71).

In the New Testament the disciples of Jesus saw a certain blind man's suffering as the result of some sin in his life or his parents (John 9:1–3), but they were wrong. Jesus repeatedly destroyed the prevailing Jewish opinion that all personal tragedy and loss could be traceable to some specific sin.

When the tower of Siloam fell on eighteen people killing them, Jesus asked the crowds who were gathered around him, "Do you think they were more guilty than all the others living in Jerusalem? I tell you, no!" (Luke 13:4–5).

In the second place, even if there is some dark sin in your closet, it does not necessarily follow that infertility is the result. One only has to look at some who are "mothers" to know that there is often no correlation between sinfulness and infertility. Prostitutes, lascivious teenagers, and abusive mothers are often allowed to conceive, while many virtuous women remain childless.

It must be granted that it is possible the Holy Spirit may convict some of us and lead us to conclude that our infertility may be the result of some grave offense against our God. If so, hopefully we will be able to bring the sin before the Savior and leave it at the cross. The forgiveness of God as it centers in the redemptive work of Jesus Christ is real, magnificent, and liberating. "If we confess our sins, he is faithful and just and will forgive us our sins and purify us from all unrighteousness" (1 John 1:9).

For the vast majority of us, however, the inclination to search for some specific shortcoming which can explain our infertility is misguided, self-defeating, destructive, and wrong. I want to hasten to add that in Scripture itself there is no indication that all or even most who suffered infertility were people who were experiencing the results of God's anger. Indeed, some of the most righteous people pictured in the Bible were people who suffered infertility. One would be hard-pressed to prove that God made Abraham and Sarah infertile because he was angry with them, or that Hannah (1 Sam. 1:1–20) couldn't have a child because she was immoral, or that Zechariah and Elizabeth were barren because they were such great sinners (Luke 1:5–25). On the contrary, these were people of great faith and righteousness. Abraham is the father of believers and of him it is said, "Against all hope, Abraham in hope believed and so became the father of many nations, just as it had been said to him" (Rom. 4:18). And of Zechariah and Elizabeth it is said, "Both of them were upright in the sight of God, observing all the Lord's commandments and regulations blamelessly" (Luke 1:6).

Many infertile couples generate a lot of bad theological thinking and a great deal of unnecessary suffering in their lives by assuming that somehow their infertility is a consequence of some shortcoming. There are two other reasons that can be suggested for the fact that God allows people to suffer and neither of them has anything to do with sin.

To strengthen us for greater faith and service

Judith Stigger in her book, *Coping with Infertility*, touches on this possibility when she says:

> From this viewpoint, infertility is not an indication of sin, but rather a tool employed by God to prepare His people for some future task—perhaps to steel their trust in and resolve to obey God's commands, or perhaps to increase their compassion for and responsiveness to the suffering of others (p. 93).

Though Stigger questions this possibility herself, I do not. There is all too much evidence in the Bible that suffering can serve this kind of purpose.

Perhaps the foremost example is to be found in the life of our Lord. One day Jesus was led by the Spirit into the desert (Matt. 4:1–11). During the next forty days, without food and facing the powerful temptations of Satan, he suffered. What was the purpose of it all?

This wilderness temptation was at the very beginning of Christ's public ministry. The Father was preparing his Son for the task before him. Jesus was getting a foretaste of what Satan intended to throw at him. Having met that first challenge, he was made stronger to face what lay ahead.

We see this same kind of strengthening purpose behind the suffering that Jesus endured in Gethsemane the night before the cross. During those long, awful hours when his sweat became as drops of blood, Jesus suffered, but in it he was strengthened to face the much greater suffering that would engulf him the next day on Calvary.

Much of the suffering we endure is meant to strengthen us. It is meant to increase our faith and make us turn more and more to the only source of strength. It is meant to refine us as gold is refined by fire (1 Peter 1:7). The Bible contains many references to this kind of suffering. Paul in Romans 5:3–5 declares, "We also rejoice in our sufferings, because we know that suffering produces perseverance; perseverance, character; and character, hope." And James in chapter 1:2–4 of his letter adds, "Consider it pure joy, my brothers, whenever you face trials of many kinds, because you know that the testing of your faith develops perseverance. Perseverance must finish its work so that you may be mature and complete, not lacking anything."

Personally, Sylvia and I know that our infertility struggle has helped us to grow spiritually. It has helped us to grow in our prayer life, for we have come to realize how utterly dependent we are on God. It has helped us in our trust, for we know that the God who has helped us resolve our infertility struggle will see us through the rest of life

as well. It has helped us grow in our sensitivity to the
suffering of others, for our infertility has led us into contact with many others who have an infertility problem
and who have not yet reached the point of resolution.

To glorify God

In our suffering, God's name can be honored. Jesus indicated this as a reason for some human suffering in the
incident briefly referred to earlier in this chapter, the healing of a certain man born blind (John 9:1–3). As the story
unfolds, Jesus and his disciples encounter the blind man
and his disciples ask Jesus, "Who sinnned, this man or
his parents, that he was born blind?" Jesus replies, "Neither this man nor his parents sinned, *but this happened
so that the work of God might be displayed in his life*
(italics added)." This man's suffering became the means
of displaying God's power, greatness, and compassion.

It is apparent that Job was allowed to suffer as well (at
least in part) in order that God's name and honor might
be vindicated in the face of Satan's insinuations. In the
opening chapter of the Book of Job, Satan had snidely
suggested that the only reason Job was "a blameless and
upright man" was that God was protecting him from all
trial and tragedy. "Stretch out your hand," said Satan,
"and strike everything he has, and he will surely curse
you to your face" (vs. 11). Satan was insulting God and
Job. To prove Satan wrong and to vindicate his faithful
servant Job, God allowed Job to suffer.

Perhaps your infertility is not because you have been
guilty of something, but because of God's grace you have
become a faithful servant like Job. As you suffer in faith,
you are bringing honor to God. Could it be that the person
you work with has seen you bear your pain in dignity and
trust, and has been moved to seek the God who has given
you so much grace? Maybe your fellow Christians have
been moved to praise God as they see your strength in the

face of trial. God can use adversity to bring honor to his name and the possibilities are endless.

At this point you may be wondering, "Where do I fit in? Is my infertility problem the result of some past grave offense? Have I been allowed to suffer because God wants to strengthen me and help me grow, or does God want to use my suffering to bring honor to him? How can I be sure of the reason?"

The answer is that most of us will never know for sure. We will probably never know exactly why God has allowed infertility to be a part of our lives. We may want an explanation—thinking that if we only knew what God's plan was, the suffering would be easier to take. We may ask for an explanation, making our "Why" question a regular part of our prayer life. But in the end most of our whys remain unanswered; the heavens remain silent. The reasons for it all remain hidden in the shadows.

God does not owe us an explanation for the suffering in our lives. Many of us tend to think he does. Joni Eareckson felt this way about God following the tragic diving accident in which she was paralyzed. Now a familiar Christian author and speaker she has these insightful comments about her earlier view of God:

> What a low view of my Master and Creator I had held all these years! How could I have dared to assume that almighty God owed me explanations! Did I think that because I had done God the "favor" of becoming a Christian, He must now check things out with me? Was the Lord of the universe under obligation to show me how the trials of every human being fit into the tapestry of life? Had I never read Deuteronomy 29:29: "There are secrets the Lord your God has not revealed to us" (LB)?
>
> What made me think that even if He explained all His ways to me I would be able to understand them? It would be like pouring million-gallon truths into my one-ounce brain. Why, even the great apostle Paul admitted that, though never in despair, he was often perplexed (2 Cor. 4:8). Hadn't God said, "For as the heavens are higher than

the earth, so are ... my thoughts (higher) than your thoughts" (Isa. 55:9)? Didn't one Old Testament author write, "As you do not know the path of the wind, or how the body is formed in a mother's womb, so you cannot understand the work of God, the Maker of all things" (Eccl. 11:5 NIV)? In fact, the whole book of Ecclesiastes was written to convince people like me that only God holds the keys to unlocking the mysteries of life and that He's not loaning them all out! "He has also set eternity in the hearts of men; yet they cannot fathom what God has done from beginning to end" (Eccl. 3:11 NIV).

If God's mind was small enough for me to understand, He wouldn't be God! How wrong I had been (Eareckson & Estes, *A Step Further*, p. 171).

Personally, I do not think it is appropriate for Christians to dwell overlong on the "Why." For it makes little ultimate difference to the Christian why God has allowed us to be infertile. This can be said because we have such a wonderful God, that whatever he allows the Christian to suffer, he transforms by his divine chemistry into our good and his glory.

The ability and power of God to transform the suffering of our lives—whatever its source—into our ultimate good is one aspect of the beautiful doctrine of providence. A historic Christian creed summarizes providence in a very personal way when it declares that those who know God may say in faith:

> I trust him so much that I do not doubt
>   he will provide
>   whatever I need
>   for body and soul,
>   and he will turn to my good
>   whatever adversity he sends me
>   in this sad world.
> He is able to do this because he is almighty God;
> he desires to do this because he is a faithful Father.
>   (The Heidelberg Catechism, Q. 26)

Infertility and Prayer

Of all the dimensions of the infertility struggle, none perhaps is so disturbing as the desolate feeling of being alone. It seems at times as if no one understands, no one cares, no one knows the pain. Even one's husband or wife does not understand.

In the days of the Old Testament, Hannah certainly felt this sense of human isolation. She was infertile and she was alone (1 Sam. 1:1–20). She received no understanding from Peninnah, her husband's other wife. Peninnah kept belittling Hannah for her failure to conceive. She also received little real understanding from her husband Elkanah whose reaction to Hannah's grief was to suggest that what she was going through wasn't that bad: "Why are you weeping. . . . Don't I mean more to you than ten sons?" (1 Sam. 1:8). His heart was probably in the right place, but he simply did not realize the depth of her pain. The clergy of that day also failed to properly understand her situation. Misinterpreting her anguished cries to the Lord, Eli, the priest, accused her of being drunk.

From a human point of view, Hannah had to bear her infertility alone. As one pastor has put it in a recent article: "The human responses to Hannah's problem were almost totally negative. She was surrounded by a taunting rival, a bungling husband, and an insensitive priest."

But Hannah was not alone. She poured out her soul to the Lord. She prayed to the One who always understands, the One who is always sensitive to our needs, the One who never bungles, the One who never taunts us. Hannah prayed to God.

Hannah's prayer to God was not some neat, formula prayer. Her words did not flow from her mouth with the ease of melted butter. Her prayer did not contain the well-polished phrases and pious clichés that plague so many of our prayers. Hannah's plea was from her heart and soul. The infertile Christian couple can learn a lot from Hannah's prayer. As the pastor referred to earlier states:

> Prayer is first of all the honest opening up of our heart to God. We need not worry whether that is okay or not. Isn't it true that God knows us inside and out? He sees us as we are and as we feel. Nothing is hidden from his sight. Why not openly talk to God about everything that fills our heart? Our hearts are enormous reservoirs of joys and disappointments, of unanswered questions and unfulfilled wishes, of hopes and despair. Our certainties are often plagued by doubts, our joys dampened by anxiety. God knows! To pray is to be candid before God's face, not to tell God what to do, but to open one's heart to him in self-disclosure (M. DeVries, *The Banner*, 1/8/83, p. 23).

Hannah was certainly not alone in making her infertility a matter of prayer. Abraham more than once made his continuing childless condition a matter for prayer with God (Gen. 15:1–4; 17:18). When the angel came to declare to Zechariah the good news that he and Elizabeth would have a child, the angel said, "Do not be afraid, Zechariah; your prayer has been heard. Your wife Elizabeth will bear you a son . . ." (Luke 1:13). We are told that "Isaac prayed to the Lord on behalf of his wife [Rebekah], because she was barren" (Gen. 25:21).

This strongly suggests that infertile Christian couples should very much make their infertility a matter of continuing, honest, heartfelt prayer to God. The evidence is clear that God hears such prayers and in mercy has granted the requests his infertile sons and daughters have made. "The prayer of a righteous man [or woman] is powerful and effective" (James 5:16).

But please be ready for surprises! God's answer to our prayers may not be what we expect or hope for. God does things in his own way and according to his own timetable, not ours. Sometimes God's answer to an earnest prayer

is "Yes," sometimes it is "No," and sometimes it is "Wait."
But whatever God's answer is, it is always right.

God never promises that he will remove all suffering
from us. He does promise us that we will never have to
suffer alone.

9

What's Right—What's Wrong?

John

Louise Brown, the world's first "test tube" baby, was born on July 25, 1978. Newspapers everywhere heralded the event as a great scientific breakthrough. Instantly new hope surged for infertile couples around the world. Questions arose as well. The "test tube" baby technique was possible, but was it right?

Actually, ethical questions concerning some forms of infertility treatment have been around a lot longer than baby Louise. For decades doctors have been treating infertility patients with AIH (artificial insemination with husband's sperm) or AID (artificial insemination with donor's sperm), and for decades Christians have been struggling with the question "Is it right?"

"Have you ever thought about trying artificial insemination?" the doctor asked. The question startled us. "No, we haven't," I finally blurted out, "Why?" "Well," he hesitated, "I think that is your best hope. It can be done with your sperm or with that of a donor."

Suddenly our physician had presented us with an enormous decision to make. We wanted to reach our goal of having a baby, but was this the route we had to take to get there? Would this be honoring to God? Was the use of artificial insemination going a step too far?

Those concerns are admittedly somewhat vague, but they were nonetheless real to us. We have not been alone. Intuitively many couples feel that something may be wrong with the artificial insemination process, but they do not know what it is. This same type of powerfully emotive but imprecise hesitation is found among many infertile Christians when faced with some of the more avant-garde means of biotechnical parenting.

Unfortunately little has been written specifically for infertile couples to help them come to grips with the ethical issues that such current treatments have raised. We hope this chapter will help to fill that void and enable Christian infertile couples to sort out in a constructive, biblical way some of the complex ethical issues involved.

In order to clarify these ethical issues a concise definition of terms and a description of procedures is necessary.

Defining Terms and Describing Procedures

Artificial Insemination

Artificial insemination involves the injection of sperm into the vagina or uterus by artificial means rather than by normal intercourse. There are three types of artificial insemination:

AIH, insemination with the husband's semen

AID, insemination with a donor's semen

IUI, insemination with semen (either husband's or donor's) that has been "washed" so that sperm can be put directly into the uterus (intrauterine insemination).

Though insemination is a simple procedure, it will help very little if other causes for infertility exist. For this reason all other factors should be ruled out first.

The technique of insemination by AID or AIH is simple. The man collects the semen by masturbating into a clean container which does not need to be sterile. The specimen is brought to the doctor's office for insertion into the woman's vagina. If AID is used, the specimen is from an anonymous donor or through a sperm bank.

If the husband's sperm count is low, the doctor may instruct him to collect only the first part of his ejaculate for AIH, because the first part of the ejaculate usually contains the greatest concentration of sperm.

Occasionally, however, the last part of the ejaculate will contain more sperm. Through tests done on the sperm, a doctor can determine which portion of the ejaculate is best in an individual case.

The technique—AIH, AID. The doctor places a special plastic cup, with a tube on one side, over the cervix. The collected semen is squirted through the tube and into the cup. A small plastic bead is used to plug the tube to keep the semen from escaping.

The cervical cup keeps the semen at the cervical opening and allows the sperm to swim into the cervical mucus and then into the uterus. Inseminations can be done without the cup, but most doctors prefer to use it.

The technique—IUI. Intrauterine insemination (IUI) is a relatively new technique for the treatment of infertility. This procedure involves the insertion of washed sperm (from husband or donor) directly into a woman's uterus. How likely it is that a woman will become pregnant with this technique is not yet known, but many women who had not conceived with other procedures have become pregnant with IUI. Although there may be other reasons found for the use of IUI in the future, many physicians now are trying IUI for the following problems:

Husband has a low sperm count, poor sperm motility, small volume of semen, excessive volume of semen, or semen that is too sticky.

Wife has cervical mucus in which sperm are not surviving: "bad" Sims-Huhner (postcoital, PK) test.

Pregnancy is not resulting when there is no obvious cause for infertility, or when the cause for infertility seems to be corrected but pregnancy does not occur, as when a woman is taking clomiphene and having regular ovulation but without subsequent pregnancy.

Husband has retrograde ejaculation (see glossary).

Intrauterine insemination (IUI) is performed in the following manner.

The semen is allowed to liquefy or is drawn back and forth through a needle to make it liquefy.

The semen is then mixed in a test tube with some tissue culture media, a liquid that is normally used to grow human or animal tissues in the laboratory. This fluid is spun on a centrifuge. Since the sperm are heavier than the other contents of this mixture, they go to the bottom of the tube. The fluid on top of the sperm is suctioned off and discarded, and more tissue culture fluid is put on top of the sperm. The contents are mixed up again and the process repeated.

A small amount of tissue culture media is then added to the now well-washed sperm, and the tube is shaken.

This solution, which now contains all the sperm, is gently squirted directly into the woman's uterus. The uterus does not react to the tissue-culture media and washed-sperm mixture in the negative way it reacts to semen, although some women will have mild cramping with IUI.

I normally do this procedure two times each month, as close to the time of ovulation as possible. The actual insemination is a simple procedure, both for the doctor and for the patient. It usually causes no more discomfort than a regular pelvic exam, although it does take time to allow for washing of the sperm.

Positive aspects of the procedure, other than the fact that it does not hurt, are that as far as we can tell now there are few complications, and some patients for whom there was "nothing left to try" are now getting pregnant using IUI.

In vitro fertilization—IVF

The procedure is theoretically fairly simple. It has been found that a woman who has IVF done is more likely to become pregnant if she can have three embryos put into her uterus with IVF. Normally a woman's ovaries produce only one egg a month. To make her ovaries develop more than one egg in a given month, an IVF patient receives Pergonal or a combination of clomiphene and Pergonal, starting soon after her period begins. Some combination of these drugs are given daily until the ovaries contain two, three, or more healthy appearing follicles (cysts).

When the follicles have developed properly, as measured by repeated ultrasound observations and repeated blood estrogen tests, each one of them usually contains a healthy egg. When these eggs seem to be at maturity and just before the body ovulates on its own, a laparoscopy is done. At laparoscopy the doctor inserts a needle into each follicle separately, applies suction, and draws the follicular fluid with its egg out of the ovary and into a separate container for each egg.

After a period of time varying from a few minutes to a few hours, a solution containing sperm is placed with each egg in its dish. Fertilization occurs in those dishes. The doctors can tell the next morning if the eggs have been fertilized.

After the embryos (the eggs that are fertilized) have grown for two or three days, they are drawn into a thin plastic tube. A speculum is put into the woman's vagina, just as with a pelvic exam, and the tube with the embryos is painlessly inserted through the cervix into the uterus. The embryos are gently pushed into the cavity of the uterus.

If the embryos stay in the uterus and continue their growth, pregnancy is established and nine months later a baby (or babies) is born. Even though more than one embryo may be placed in the uterus, all of them do not usually survive.

GIFT

A recent adaption of IVF is a procedure called gamete intrafallopian transfer (GIFT). This procedure, in most programs, is limited to women with one or two normal fallopian tubes. GIFT is done exactly like IVF through the point at which the eggs have been removed from the woman's ovaries. Instead of being allowed to wake from anesthesia at this point, however, the woman is kept asleep for a short additional time. While she remains on the operating table, eggs and sperm are drawn into a thin plastic tube. This tube is brought into the operating room and inserted through the incision made for the needle that was used to retrieve the eggs. The tip of this plastic tube is threaded into one of the fallopian tubes and eggs and sperm are squirted into the fallopian tube. The procedure is repeated with the other fallopian tube. The instruments are removed and the incision is closed. The woman is allowed to wake up and go home, hopefully to become pregnant. No other treatment is necessary, except perhaps the use of progesterone shots or progesterone vaginal suppositories until she knows whether or not she is pregnant. With GIFT, pregnancy occurs spontaneously in the woman's fallopian tube, the place where pregnancy normally occurs. The embryos then pass into the uterus where in the normal fashion they either become a growing pregnancy or pass on out as a very early miscarriage. Preliminary studies indicate a 30-percent pregnancy rate with this procedure. It is somewhat less expensive and less time-consuming than IVF.

Three methods of achieving pregnancy that go beyond the regular IVF and GIFT techniques are: (1) *Frozen embryos.* Unused IVF embryos are frozen and "banked" for use in subsequent months if pregnancy is not achieved. (2) *Embryo transfers.* Embryos conceived in one woman are "washed out" of her uterus and transplanted into the uterus of an infertile woman. (3) *Surrogate mothers.* A woman will contract with a couple to bear and deliver their child, which is conceived either by embryo transfer from a woman who, for example, has ovaries but no uterus, or by insemination of the surrogate's egg with the husband's sperm.

Having defined and described the procedures, it is now necessary to turn to the ethical and moral issues involved in each of these procedures.

Looking at Ethical and Moral Issues

Artificial insemination with husband's sperm (AIH)

There appear to be only a few ethicists, non-Christian or Christian, who have significant reservations about AIH. Some of the more conservative Catholic ethicists contend that AIH separates the unitive and procreative aspects of human sexuality which intrinsically belong together.

A few non-Catholic ethicists also have a problem with AIH on similar grounds that it depersonalizes an essentially human act. Such an ethicist is Dr. Leon Kass who asks:

Is there possibly some wisdom in that mystery of nature which joins the pleasure of sex, the communication of love, and desire for children in the very activity by which we continue the chain of human existence? . . . Before we embark on "New Beginnings in Life" we should consider the meaning of the union between sex, love, and procreation and the meaning and consequences of its cleavage (*The New Genetics and the Future of Man*, pp. 53-54).

One of the associated problems raised with AIH is that it necessarily entails masturbation. This has caused concern to some couples, particularly those in the Roman Catholic communion.

However, most theologians and ethicists have very little problem with AIH. This includes a number of Catholic writers who argue that the "partners express their love regularly by intercourse which they would render fertile if they could, but since they cannot, they use an artificial process to achieve their legitimate purpose."

Even if such theologians have a problem with masturbation generally, they do not when it involves treatment of infertility. It is argued that there is an essential moral difference between masturbation as an act whose object is sexual gratification and the same physical act whose object is to allow a husband and wife to conceive a baby.

Personally I came to have little ethical difficulty with AIH and we did in fact pursue this course of treatment for our infertility—albeit unsuccessfully. It was not a particularly pleasant experience, but I never felt it was immoral. I agree that ideally sex, love, and procreation belong together in the unitive act of a husband and wife. Where that does not achieve a pregnancy, I can see no valid objection to AIH. I do not see AIH as separation of the couple's love for each other but rather as a result of that love. In AIH the child is in fact conceived as the fruit of the union between a man and his wife. The artificial means merely assist a natural process which for one reason or another is not working.

Artificial insemination with donor sperm (AID)

The first concern that AID raises is the possibility that it may be tantamount to committing adultery. In some countries there are laws which treat AID as adultery.

Adultery involves an act of intercourse or at least—in terms of Matthew 5:28—lustful desire. But AID involves no such act of intercourse or lust.

Some people have a more serious objection to AID (as

well as some of the other procedures mentioned below). They feel it is intrinsically wrong because it inevitably and undeniably involves a third party in the marriage relationship, though in a non-adulterous way.

As Dr. E. G. Postma, a Christian obstetrician, comments in an article on AID:

> When one understands the "one flesh" concept in mar-riage as a holy sexual unity, from which, in normal sit-uations and at certain times, new individuals may find their beginnings, then the active insinuation of another individual's active genetic potential and personal history into that unity seems to be disruptive. The woman is now engaged with someone else (anonymously and sexlessly) in bringing a new life into that unity. The female part of the one-flesh unity is active in unilaterally conceiving, carrying, and delivering one whom God ordains to be naturally the result of the unity. ... When one of the partners uses his or her individual portion of the one-flesh sexuality to "father" or "mother" a new individual outside of their particular male-female unity, it seems to me, in that instance, to be destroying the one-flesh con-cept of that partnership (*The Banner*, 2/11/77, p. 9).

To the objection that adoption involves the same kind of disruption, Postma argues that, on the contrary, in the case of adoption "The one flesh concept remains inviolate. Both prospective parents stand in the same relationship to the adopted child."

Perhaps the most vague and yet most troublesome issue of all is the question of where the technological process involved in AID will finally lead. The Christian cannot help but be conscious of the concern that such biotech-nological parenting can lead to what has been called a "sperm-bank mentality." Already there are such banks (e.g., the Nobel Sperm Bank in Southern California) in which samples of sperm from Nobel prize winners are stored and made available for insemination. The sperm-bank mentality presupposes that superior traits can be programmed and dictated. This too raises a host of questions for society and for Christians. Should any couple who wants to have "superior" children be allowed to make use of such a repository? And what qualities are judged to be superior? Is intelligence the number-one superior quality? As George F. Will points out, "The qualities that seem to make life livable—compassion, courage, magnanimity—do not seem to figure in the bank's scheme of things" (*Argus Leader*, July 22, 1982). If Christians consciously—and who can blame them—choose "superior" quality sperm for their prospective AID (or in vitro) child, are they not supporting the sperm-bank mentality?

To the above concerns can also be added the following potential problems inherent in the use of AID. Although these potential problems are not strictly ethical in nature, they do entail considerations which the Christian infertile couple should take into account.

Artificial insemination by donor is an accepted medical practice and legal problems are fairly rare, but they do occasionally arise. Twenty-five states now have laws recognizing AID babies as the legitimate children of the mother and her husband—providing that the husband was willing to give consent to the procedure. In the remaining states those who use this procedure are in a legal no-man's land if litigation arises (e.g., the donor goes to court to obtain parental rights for his progeny or a couple obtains a divorce and the husband refuses to pay child support to his ex-wife on the grounds that he is not really the father of their AID-conceived child).[1]

There is the potential for unwitting incest. It is conceivable, for example, that a young man conceived by AID

1. Presently most courts are following a precedent established by a California court in *The People vs. Sorenson* (1968). A judge in that case ruled that a husband who had given consent for his wife to be inseminated with a donor was liable for child support even though the couple was separated and divorced. Indications are that most rulings have relied heavily on the consent forms both partners signed after the AID procedure was carefully explained to them (B. E. Menning, *Contemporary OB/GYN*, Oct. 1981, p. 6).

would decide to marry a young woman who is biologically his half-sister because she was also conceived by AID and born to another couple. This may not be as remote a possibility as many assume.

Will a husband and wife be able to psychologically accept the child as their own even though the child is not biologically the husband's? As Judith Stigger writes in her book, *Coping with Infertility:*

> Artificial insemination requires an emotional adjustment especially for the man. The baby is biologically hers but not his, as opposed to adoption where both spouses are on equal footing. The risk is that for a man and woman who have not come to terms with his infertility, the baby may become emotionally hers but not his (p. 76).

To help overcome this problem some physicians mix the husband's sperm with the sperm of a donor. This provides the infertile couple with some reason to believe that the child is biologically theirs.

We assume that most physicians inform their patients and seek their permission before utilizing this procedure. Unfortunately the doctor who initially treated us with AIH was not that candid.

Before actually undergoing AIH Sylvia thought it wise to ask, "Doctor, will I be inseminated only with John's sperm?" The physician in question looked a little nonplussed. "Well, no," he said, "I was going to mix John's sperm with that of a fertile donor." When we both looked at each other; he added somewhat defensively, "If we use John's sperm alone, I do not recommend artificial insemination. John's motility level is questionable. By mixing John's sperm with a donor, you will never know for sure who the father is. If it gives you greater peace of mind to think that John is the father, you may certainly do so."

This is not accepted practice. Any time a doctor is going to inseminate a woman with sperm from a source other than her own husband, that should be clearly explained to them. They should sign a permission form for this donor insemination. It makes no difference whether or not the husband's sperm is also used, the procedure is still artificial insemination with donor sperm and should be handled as such.

There is also the problem of confidentiality. The couple initially has to decide who, if any, among their close friends and relatives they should tell, and ultimately whether they should tell their offspring. The couple may, in fact, decide to tell no one, not even the child who has been born to them via AID. This does not necessarily solve all the problems. One possible scenario might involve a child growing to maturity and developing an illness or injury in which the medical history of the family becomes critically important. It may then be eminently embarrassing or even traumatic for him to learn that only half of his family's medical history is valid because he is not genetically related to the father.

Is the procedure known as AID a legitimate option for Christians? I am not prepared to say that the above objections and problems are of sufficient ethical weight to prohibit AID from a Christian point of view. If it is for the purpose of allowing a married, infertile couple to achieve the child they so desperately want, and if both partners have conscientiously and seriously explored the implications and questions involved, I would not judge them immoral or unethical.

Personally, however, I could not involve myself in such a process. The reason for this is perhaps psychological as much as ethical. I simply do not know if I could accept the fact that my wife was impregnated by another man's sperm. The ethical and legal considerations, however, do play a role in my personal refusal to have a child via AID.

For I cannot escape the gnawing conclusion that AID does take technology out of the covenant of marriage and in some sense may be jeopardizing the oneness of marriage and family or may pose a threat to the personal identity of the child.

If a Christian infertile couple came to me for my advice on whether or not to pursue AID, I would try to help them carefully consider the ethical, psychological, and legal issues involved and leave it up to their informed Christian consciences to make the final decision. And if such a couple, after prayerful and careful reflection, wanted to pursue this process, I would help them secure the best medical care available.

It seems to me that adultery involves the physical coming together of two people in sexual union outside of marriage. The transfer of another man's sperm to the wife of an infertile man, since it does not involve the third person in the marriage physically, would therefore not seem to me to be adultery.

Donor inseminations have been a part of my infertility practice for many years. I have prayerfully considered the biblical, moral, and ethical aspects of this procedure and am comfortable performing it.

It might interest couples who feel AID is right for them to know that I have not had any couples express any regret about having undergone the AID procedure. Several couples have returned to have a second child using AID. Many of these women are long-term patients and I am not aware of any problems that developed for them or their husbands after using AID to help them have a child.

If, after the AID procedure has been thoroughly discussed, a husband or wife (or both) is uncomfortable

with using it, that couple should not have the AID
procedure done, regardless of the intensity of their desire
to achieve pregnancy.

Intrauterine insemination (IUI)

Intrauterine insemination raises new hope for some infertile couples and poses no new ethical considerations.
Granted, IUI does involve manipulation of the sperm, but
most ethicists have never considered tampering with
sperm to be the moral equivalent of tampering with an
embryo—one is human life and the other is not.

In my judgment the ethical considerations of IUI are
the same as those which were discussed in connection
with AIH and AID.

In vitro fertilization (IVF)

In vitro fertilization is becoming increasingly available
to infertile couples in this country. At the end of 1985
there were approximately 120 IVF clinics in the U.S. The
availability of these clinics will cause many Christian couples to face the question, "Is in vitro an option for us as
Christians?"

I think it can be. If this option were pursued, however,
my strong personal, ethical inclination is that it be intra-
marital (i.e., husband's sperm—wife's egg). Theoretically
there could be five people intimately involved in parenting a child via the in vitro process—a woman who donates her egg, a man who donates his sperm, a woman
who agrees to use her womb as host for the embryo, and
the recipient couple.

My cautious acceptance of in vitro also presupposes
that all of the embryos are implanted into the uterus of
the infertile woman undergoing treatment. Personally I
am of the conviction that human life begins at fertilization with the union of the egg and sperm. From that moment something unique has been formed, an unrepeatable
combination of genes resulting in a unique individual.

The doctors involved in St. David's Community Hospital's in vitro program (which I helped to establish and actively practice in) have a very high regard for the embryo, as do many in vitro clinics. We transfer all embryos back to the mother, except for one specific situation.

If more than one sperm fertilizes an egg, the resulting embryo has too many chromosomes. This condition is totally incompatible with life. As a matter of fact, most of these embryos fail to survive more than a few days. If they did grow in a woman's uterus, some might survive for a few months before they were miscarried. Were a woman to deliver a child that was the result of this type of pregnancy, it would not be able to survive after birth. Therefore, since such a polyspermic embryo could cause the loss of a normal fetus that might be growing in the uterus with it, we do not transfer a polyspermic embryo back to the uterus.

This is the only abnormality that can be detected in embryos in an IVF program since embryos are transferred back into the uterus so soon. Therefore, IVF cannot be used to select healthy or abnormal fetuses.

If you are a Christian infertile couple contemplating in vitro fertilization as a legitimate Christian option, I would urge you to consider a couple of facts before you pursue this approach. They have nothing to do with the rightness or wrongness of the matter, but you ought to be aware of them in making a wise decision about in vitro.

In vitro is expensive. Most clinics require a fee of $3,000 to $5,000 per attempt. Some fees are reportedly as high as $10,000. One New York couple who tried seven times at the Norfolk in vitro clinic before finally achieving pregnancy, figure the total cost was $80,000. Currently only a few insurance companies have been willing to assume expenses because they view IVF as being an experimental procedure.

The chances of achieving pregnancy through in vitro,
although improving, are slim.

The success rate is about 20 percent each time it is
done. This means if a couple has IVF twice, they have a
40-percent chance of achieving pregnancy.

About half of the 120 IVF clinics in the United States
have not reported a single pregnancy. Some of these
clinics are set up in an excellent way medically but have
not taken care of enough patients yet to report a
pregnancy. Other older clinics though seemingly
organized in an excellent way have not had any
successful pregnancies.

It is most important, therefore, that a couple find a
good IVF clinic, either one that they are confident is
organized in a medically expert way and has the promise
of future pregnancies occurring, or a clinic that has had at
least one baby born as a result of the clinic's IVF
procedures. Unfortunately some IVF clinics are not totally
honest about their statistics. Those clinics will claim that
they have a high pregnancy rate but they include all their
patients who had "chemical pregnancies"—a positive
pregnancy test soon after the IVF procedure but before
the woman has missed a period. Such a situation is not
considered an IVF pregnancy by totally honest clinics.

Frozen embryos

Headlines around the world have recently announced
the birth of babies who were born from IVF programs that
used frozen embryos. This is a very attractive possibility
from the purely technical point of view but has major
moral and ethical problems. At IVF laparoscopy it is
common to retrieve more than four eggs. However, putting
more than four embryos back into the woman's uterus
does not improve her chance of achieving pregnancy. If
the extra eggs could be fertilized, frozen, and saved till
the next month, the embryos could be thawed and

inserted into the woman's uterus without repeating *any* of
the IVF process. And, as a matter of fact, this is being
done in a few centers around the world. But it is a very
inefficient process. Thousands of embryos have been
frozen, thawed, and placed in women's uteri but only a
few successful pregnancies have occurred. It will take
years to know if these children are physically and mentally
normal. The following discussion is quiet pertinent to the
issue of frozen embryos.

As attractive as frozen embryology may be, it presents
real ethical and moral problems. For one thing, it is estimated that 30 to 50 percent of the embryos do not live
through the deep-freezing process. For those of us who
believe that human life begins at conception, this loss of
life is intolerable.

In addition, the problem of unused embryos becomes
acute. If the infertile couple conceives and gives birth by
means of the frozen embryo route, they will be faced with
a very great temptation to simply allow the leftovers to
be discarded.

To complicate the matter further, suppose that something fatal happens to the couple before their embryos
can be implanted. In such an event the frozen embryos,
the nascent human lives they have left on ice, will be
entering uncharted legal and moral waters.

Nothing illustrates this more dramatically than the well-
publicized story of the late Mario and Elsa Del Rios. In
1984 this couple died in a tragic plane crash in Chile leaving their orphaned embryos in a freezer in Melbourne,
Australia. Whose embryos were they? Who should decide
what would become of them? The government? The ex-
ecutors of the Rios' estate? Who?

While deeply conscious of the benefits of frozen embryology, I am also deeply concerned about the loss of
human life and the moral, legal quagmire this procedure

entails. In good conscience I must demur from recommending this option for the Christian infertile couple.

I strongly agree with this conclusion.

GIFT

The new procedure known as GIFT (gamete intrafallopian transfer) is a very appealing adaptation of IVF. Because the eggs and sperm are inserted directly into the fallopian tubes, GIFT brings the process one step closer to the way pregnancy occurs naturally (i.e. in the fallopian tube of the mother-to-be). GIFT also precludes the possibility that any unneeded embryos will be discarded.

Surrogate motherhood

Surrogate motherhood inevitably raises many of the concerns and problems already addressed, but surrogate motherhood complicates the matter in that the host mother (i.e., the woman in whom the sperm of the prospective father has been implanted) must carry the baby to term and then deliver the baby to the recipient couple. Unlike AID in which the donor never sees or experiences in any way the life he helped to bring into the world, the surrogate mother lives with the fetus for nine months. Since the bonding process (the process by which a mother becomes emotionally attached to the baby) begins long before birth, many surrogate mothers have become emotionally attached to the babies they are asked to relinquish.

Another type of problem can develop if the resultant baby is malformed or mentally impaired. In such cases there is a real possibility that no one wants the child or accepts responsibility for him or her. The lead paragraph in a *TIME* editorial (Feb. 14, 1983, p. 90) graphically presents a case in point:

Three weeks ago the nation recoiled at the story of a microcephalic child, called Baby Doe by the court, who apparently was born without parents. Judy Stiver, the surrogate mother who bore him after being artificially inseminated, claimed that Baby Doe belonged to Alexander Malahoff, who had contracted to pay Stiver $10,000 on delivery. Malahoff, who is separated from his wife, and who hoped the baby might reunite them, accepted the deformed child in the beginning, and had him baptized. Later he rejected the boy, contending Baby Doe was not his own. . . . From Baby Doe's birth on Jan. 10, he was seen and discussed as a piece of inferior merchandise, an imperfect creature come into the world as damaged goods. The mother disavowed motherhood; the father said, "not mine." Yet there was the child, frail but present. Deposited on the doorstep, he had to belong to somebody.[2]

The committed Christian infertile couple may say, "That's awful. If we pursued the route of surrogate motherhood, we would accept any baby, deformed or not." This is a noble sentiment, and hopefully true. It must be pointed out, however, that it is far easier to make such statements in the abstract than when faced with a deformed baby.

Aside from this problem, one has to face the fact that the surrogate motherhood process can very easily lead to the kind of commercialism Christians ought to deplore. Because infertile couples so desperately want a baby, and because people are naturally greedy, the "buying and selling" of babies becomes a very real possibility. Already one hears the phrases "wombs for rent" or "human embryos for sale" in connection with surrogate motherhood. And one unemployed nurse who offered to bear a child for $10,000 admitted candidly that she did it "to make some money."

2. In a strange twist to this incident, later test results showed that Malahoff was not the father. Apparently Stiver had had intercourse with her husband at about the same time she had undergone the insemination and her husband was indeed the father. Last reports have indicated that the child is now in the custody of the Stivers.

If a surrogate mother is not providing her womb out of a commercial motive but rather out of genuine love and a desire to help a distressed infertile couple, the ethics of the matter become more complicated. I personally do not recommend surrogate motherhood even if the surrogate mother is providing her services free of charge and with the most admirable of motives. I cannot evade the growing conviction that this process asks of a surrogate mother that which is morally impermissible to ask her to do: give up a child conceived in her womb and carried by her for nine months before birth.

While surrogate mothers may begin by not viewing the child they are bearing as their own, imperceptibly and inevitably many will begin to do so. One does not give up a baby as if one were discarding a set of used clothes. If a woman voluntarily gives up her child as in adoption that is fine. However, one may not ask a woman to give up a child before that child is even conceived, and that is what is required in surrogate motherhood.

> The validity of this position is born out by the fact that on several occasions already in the short time that surrogate motherhood has been available, the surrogate mother could not bring herself to release her newborn to the contracting couple. This situation is tragic for all the parties involved. It leaves a couple without a child they thought was going to be theirs, and genetically *is* the husband's child. It must also leave the surrogate mother with great emotional scars. While legally she can keep the child, she has broken a contract and greatly disappointed the couple who has a very legitimate claim to the baby.

Embryo transfer

Embryo transfer adds some new twists to the procedures already described and deserves separate treatment. Dr. Robert G. Wells, an obstetrician-gynecologist, who has written a very significant article on embryo transfer for *Christianity Today* (3/2/84, pp. 28-31) describes the process this way:

> ... sperm from the husband of an infertile wife ... is inseminated into another woman—a fertile donor. Five days after conception has taken place in the donor ... the fertilized egg is washed from her uterus ... [and] transferred back into the uterus of the infertile wife who ... delivers the baby. ... genetically one-half her husband's but one-half the egg donor's—the other woman's (p. 28).

In contrast to several of the other techniques for overcoming infertility (such as in vitro fertilization), embryo transfer has several distinct advantages. It is far less expensive, requires no surgery, can be conducted in a doctor's office, has a success rate as high as 50 percent, and perhaps most significantly of all, can give the infertile woman the emotional and psychological satisfaction, so important to many, of experiencing pregnancy and childbirth. In addition, unlike surrogate motherhood in which there is the potential for many people to know that the child has been conceived artificially, with embryo transfer that complication can be avoided.

Nevertheless, there are problems. These include many of the legal and psychological problems discussed earlier in those processes involving a third party.

Foremost among the concerns for a Christian must be the question of whether such a procedure is morally and ethically right. At this time, I would have to give a qualified "no" response to that question. As someone who believes strongly in the sanctity of human life from conception on, I have to conclude that embryo transfer involves an abortionlike procedure in which a significant number of human embryos are lost.

The first human embryo transfer was successfully achieved in April of 1983 by Drs. John Buster and Maria

Bustillo of Harbor-UCLA Medical Center. But according to reports, Drs. Bustillo and Buster were not able to transfer successfully eight of eleven fertilized ova. It is likely that some—if not all—of these fertilized ova were lost in the transfer. If so, they were in effect aborted.

It has been suggested that there is another way in which embryos will be lost. In a number of cases it is possible that the embryo will not be washed out of the donor's uterus. Such a donor will more than likely not want to carry such a "retained pregnancy" to term. An obvious option for her in today's permissive climate is to have an abortion.

As a matter of fact, most embryo transfer clinics require that the donor sign a form that she will have an abortion done if she were to become pregnant because all the embryos did not wash out of her uterus.

Some well-known theologians do not share my reservation. Lewis Smedes, a professor of ethics at Fuller Theological Seminary, in an article in *Christianity Today* (3/2/84) argues:

We should remember that the woman undergoing an abortion and the woman seeking an ovum transfer intend two different things. The woman who has an abortion intends to be rid of the fetus. The woman receiving the ovum transfer intends to gain a fetus she could not otherwise have. Her desire is precisely the opposite of a woman seeking an abortion (p. 31).

Recognizing the point that Smedes has made I, nevertheless, have to sadly conclude that embryo transfer in its present state-of-the-art application necessarily, though not intentionally, may involve the loss of human life through human manipulation. If the stage is reached in which embryo transfer will no longer involve significant loss of life—and according to reports great strides are being made in that direction—my ethical reservations would be resolved to a great extent. In the meantime, I have a great deal of sympathy and understanding for those Christian couples who may choose this route for overcoming their infertility, but I cannot recommend it.

Biblical Perspectives on the Ethical Issues

At some point in discussions on the rightness or wrongness of AID, surrogate motherhood, and other biotechnical methods of infertility treatment, some Christians will bring up biblical examples of unorthodox parenting to justify the current approaches. The biblical example of Sarai giving Hagar to Abram (later renamed Abraham) so that he could father a child is often cited. The Old Testament practice of Levirate marriage is also often mentioned. Do not these biblical precedents, it is asked, supply evidence that God may condone some fairly unusual ways for people to have children? To answer this question we need to look at the Bible carefully.

The incident with Sarai, Hagar, and Abram is recorded in Genesis 16:1–2:

> Now Sarai, Abram's wife, had borne him no children. But she had an Egyptian maidservant named Hagar; so she said to Abram, "The LORD has kept me from having children. Go, sleep with my maidservant; perhaps I can build a family through her."

It is understandable that some authors use this episode as a biblical warrant for surrogate motherhood. The example of Abram and Sarai is, however, a very unfortunate one in terms of supporting the concept of surrogate motherhood. In the first place, the context makes it clear that this was Sarai's and Abram's idea and not God's. One commentator puts it succinctly when he points out: "Sarai and Abram worked out their problem together. But this was purely human planning on their part. The Lord was not given a say." God, in fact, made it very clear in talking to Abram that the son of the promise, the son God intended Abram to have, would not be from Hagar but from Sarai, his wife (Gen. 17:15–22).

Furthermore, Hagar was not some anonymous, willing woman; she in accordance with the custom of that day became Abram's wife. She was not in the strict sense of the term a surrogate mother, for her child was conceived within the context of marriage.

Finally, it is evident that Abram's and Sarai's use of "a surrogate" resulted in a tremendous amount of turmoil and distress in Abram's family. Hagar, who was now also Abram's wife, began to look down on Sarai and despise her (Gen. 16:4). In turn, Sarai began to hate Hagar and mistreat her (Gen. 16:6). Inevitably tension began to mount between Abram and Sarai: "Then Sarai said to Abram, 'You are responsible for the wrong I am suffering' " (Gen. 16:5). The net result was a searing, bitter brokenness in Abram's family as Hagar and Ishmael, her son, are sent away into the wilderness (Gen. 21:8–21). The sad story of Abram and Hagar is not a good precedent for surrogate motherhood.

Just as the incident of Abram and Sarai is used to support the concept of surrogate motherhood, some biblical ethicists (e.g., Norman Geisler of Dallas Theological Seminary, *Ethics: Alternatives and Issues*, p. 229) use the biblical description of Levirate marriage to support the concept of AID. Such support, however, is equally debatable.

Levirate literally means "husband's brother," and it refers to the legal responsibility that fell to a brother when a married man died childless. In such cases it was the duty of the brother to take the widow as his wife. Children of this marriage were considered children of the first husband. Deuteronomy 25:5–6 gives the clearest biblical expression to the Levirate concept:

If brothers are living together and one of them dies without a son, his widow must not marry outside the family.
Her husband's brother shall take her and marry her and
fulfill the duty of a brother-in-law to her. The first son she
bears shall carry on the name of the dead brother so that
his name will not be blotted out from Israel.

The Book of Ruth shows that the custom apparently
extended even beyond the husband's brother. Apparently
(see chapter 4:1–12) an unnamed kinsman has the primary responsibility to marry Ruth, and only after he refuses, does Boaz marry her.

In Levirate marriage we do see a very beautiful expression of God's concern for childless couples. It was seen as
a curse by the Old Testament people of God to be childless
and heirless. To help lift the burden of bearing such a
stigma, as well as provide support for the widow in her
old age, God provided the Levirate process.

There is, however, one crucial difference between the
Levirate practice and AID. When a child was born via the
Levirate approach, that child was born in the context and
covenant of marriage. It may have been polygamous marriage, to be sure, but it was nonetheless marriage. As
J. Kirby Anderson states in *Genetic Engineering*: "The unitive and procreative aspects of marriage remained in-
tact" (p. 40). The Levirate law was very explicit that the
brother take his dead brother's wife to be his wife! It was
not the case that the brother simply had sex with his
deceased brother's wife, and thereby helped her obtain
children; he married her.

In my judgment, those couples who attempt to support
AID by appealing to the biblical concept of Levirate marriage are not doing full justice to the biblical picture. I
am not hereby condemning AID; I am simply saying that
to justify AID on the basis of the Levirate practice is not
conclusive.

This chapter is certainly not the last word (or even my
last word) on the ethical and other problems related to

current biotechnical means of helping the Christian infertile couple achieve the child they so desperately want. The issues involved are very personal for me, complex, and subject to divided opinion among Christians. But I hope that my statements can add to the discussion and help some of the infertile Christian couples who struggle along with me to deal honestly with the issues raised.

There are many procedures medicine can accomplish today which should not be done. This seems particularly true in the reproductive area. We have barely seen the start of choices that will be available to us in the future. Genetic engineering, the fusion of two eggs to produce a baby, and increased emphasis on abortion of fetuses with defects are only a few of the issues we as Christians will face in the future. It is vital that the Christian community confront these moral challenges head on. We must literally put our feet down and say no to those things that are wrong.

Not to dilute what I have just said, I also think it is incumbent on us to accent those things that are morally acceptable and not be afraid to use them today just because they are new and because we are afraid of what they will lead to in the future. We need to have the moral courage to know we can and will speak up when an acceptable procedure is being perverted. We need to have the courage at that point of change to say: "It is acceptable up to this point but the proposed change is morally and ethically wrong and we will not tolerate it."

10

When Is Enough, Enough?

John and Sylvia

Hopefully, you are among the 50 to 60 percent of those couples who will eventually overcome an infertility problem. But realistically you have to face the facts. You may be among those couples, who though receiving extensive medical treatment, will experience no positive results in terms of either pregnancy or childbirth.

If so, there is one question that will need to be faced sooner or later. When is enough, enough? When should you stop active medical treatment? When should you call a halt to your determined pursuit of biological parenting? When do you redirect your focus from the infertility that has demanded so much attention for months and years and get on with the rest of your life?

It goes without saying that this is an extremely important and difficult decision to make. But it is one which some of us must make if we are not to devote our whole lives to trying to get pregnant.

It is also a very personal decision. No one can provide

135

a pat formula. The decision for each couple will be based
on factors whose importance only they can determine.

For some couples this question answers itself. Friends
of ours who were receiving treatment for infertility experienced two tubal pregnancies in a period of two years.
At first there was the possibility of reconstructive surgery
for one of the tubes, but the doctor, after studying the
situation carefully, was forced to conclude that it was a
forlorn hope. This couple could possibly pursue in vitro
fertilization, but barring the use of such biotechnical
methods, they know they will never have their own biological child.

For most couples the matter never becomes that clear.
They may continue medical treatment for years and never
be sure whether or not such treatment will eventually
result in pregnancy and childbirth.

For some the decision to stop trying may eventually
come as a result of a change point in their lives—a move
to another city, a new career, news that you have been
accepted by an adoption agency, the necessity of further
treatment, the celebration of your thirty-fifth birthday.
For others the decision may simply come as a result of a
slowly dawning awareness that enough time, energy, and
finances have been invested in the long marathon to have
biological children, and it is now time to devote personal
and financial resources elsewhere.

After enduring extensive tests (and re-tests) it was determined that John had a lower than normal sperm count
and motility level, and I had adhesions on my fallopian
tubes and a cyst on my left ovary. In the estimation of
several of our physicians, both John's problem and mine
stood a good chance of being corrected. John went on
medication and I had a laparotomy. Following my laparotomy we had raised hopes of achieving a pregnancy,
but it did not happen.

Nor did it happen when a year later we began seeing
an endocrinologist and attempted AIH. It did not happen

either, when we moved and began seeing another physician, and I went through two laparoscopies (both of which were to remove returning adhesions and drain my persistent cyst).

Through it all, each of our doctors remained optimistic that we could achieve a pregnancy, but it never happened. Consequently, we could never be sure, nor could anyone tell us, why we were not able to have a baby.

Today we are no longer seeking medical treatment, nor is achieving a pregnancy on the list of our life goals. This was not a sudden decision but a gradual one. Finally it simply all caught up with us, the passing of the years, the weariness of all the testing and charting, the expense, the pain of three operations, and the lure of more obtainable goals. If there was one clinching factor in our decision to call it quits, it was the adoption of our second child. With two children in our home, our life became filled with new challenges and blessings. We knew it was time to say, "Enough is enough."

If you find yourself in the uncomfortable position of trying to determine when enough is enough, consider the following suggestions.

Be willing to face the facts. If you have honestly given the achievement of a pregnancy your "best shot," do not hesitate to ask your doctor to sit down with you and candidly discuss your prognosis.

If you do initiate such a conversation with your physician (or if he or she initiates such a conversation) you do yourself a favor if you make it clear that you want an open and honest answer. In some cases the physician may be relieved when his or her infertility patients ask for an honest opinion. The doctor may have been looking for an opportunity to let the patients know where things really stand, but has been reluctant to do so for fear of causing hurt and disappointment.

The decision should be made by both husband and wife. This is extremely important. When the decision is not reached by mutual agreement you are providing the breeding ground for resentment ("I wish you hadn't stopped seeing Dr. Jones") or guilt ("If only I had listened to my husband and tried one more time . . .").

Do not make a hasty decision. Remember that infertility testing and treatment by its very nature involves a long, intensive, expensive process which is bound to produce anxiety and frustration. Understanding this and preparing yourselves for it at the very beginning can help you to avoid the "early drop-out syndrome." If you quit before you have really given achieving pregnancy an honest and extensive attempt, you may regret it for the rest of your lives.

Do not be afraid to change your mind. It may be that you will reach a point where you have had it. You become tired of monthly doctor's visits, huge medical fees, programmed sex. Perhaps you are discouraged because there is no pregnancy after prolonged medical care, or you simply cannot face another operation. The net result is that you terminate treatment. Fine! But do not be afraid to change your mind. In six months or a year, you may be refreshed and hopeful enough to try again. If so, do not be ashamed to call your doctor. You are not the first couple who changed their minds, neither will you be the last.

Do not be unduly influenced by others. There may be those around you, family members or close friends, who simply cannot understand why you are giving up. "How can you quit now?" they will ask, "You're only thirty-two. Why don't you give it some more time?" You as a couple must decide when enough is enough. You know your situation and experience. Do not let outside pressure push you into continuing when you have had enough.

Make this a matter of sincere prayer as you seek God's guidance and wisdom. This is mentioned last, but it is certainly not least.

11

Adoption as an Option

John and Sylvia

Not flesh of my flesh,
Nor bone of my bone,
but still miraculously
    My own.

Never forget
For a single minute:
You didn't grow under my heart,
    But in it.

                        Heyliger

    This poem on the wall of the adoption agency greeted us during our first visit. We were there for an adoption interview. For us that poem became a living reality, for we were to become the parents of two beautiful, adopted children. For us adoption has been a very positive experience. We would not trade the opportunity we have had to enjoy our two children for anything in the world.

    At about the time the infertile couple decides that

enough is enough in terms of medical treatment, they begin to explore alternatives. Adoption is number-one on the list.

My general recommendation is this: after you have had a full evaluation and have had a year of treatment without becoming pregnant, you should consider starting the adoption process.

I encourage you to continue trying to become pregnant, however, because the adoption process often requires two or more years of waiting before a child actually arrives in your home. It is possible that during this time you could become pregnant.

Adoption agencies generally do not mind if you continue your attempts to become pregnant while working with them on an adoption. If you become pregnant, you can always cancel the adoption process.

Trying to adopt a child has an additional advantage if you have been unsuccessfully trying to become pregnant for quite some time. It can be a pressure-relief valve even while you continue your infertility treatments, because you will know that one way or the other, you should have your new baby.

A doctor can be of great help, not only in working out a plan for your infertility evaluation and treatment, but also helping with the adoption process. The three of you should keep talking as you proceed through every step of the fertility evaluation and as you consider adoption.

What Does God Say About Adoption?

Surprisingly, the Bible speaks about adoption rather often. Adoption is presented as a positive, gracious act. Moses was an adoptee, as in a way was Jesus. Personally, we think that Joseph, Jesus' adoptive father, was special. There was a rare unselfishness about him. He was willing to restructure his whole life in obedience to God. He was willing to bear a sense of shame in parenting Jesus—for he alone of all men knew that Jesus was not his biological child. Joseph accepted Jesus gladly, giving him all the love, encouragement, and guidance that any father would provide for his son. We can learn a great deal from Joseph.

The greatest adoption story recorded in all the Bible is the adoption of believers into the family of God. The Living Bible puts it beautifully when it paraphrases Ephesians 1:5: "His unchanging plan has always been to adopt us into his own family by sending Jesus Christ to die for us. And he did this because he wanted to!"

Just think! God chose us to be adoptive children not because he had to, but because he wanted to. For God, this adoption process was special. In it he was able to show his great love. What a model this presents for those who want to adopt a child as their son or daughter.

For the Christian infertile couple, adoption is not "second best." It is simply the way that God in his wisdom can choose for us to be parents. Whether one becomes a parent biologically or through adoption, the fact is that children are not a right but a gift from God: "Sons are a heritage from the Lord" (Ps. 127:3). The person who becomes a parent through biologically having children has no right to sinful pride ("Look what I have been able to do"), and the one who receives a child by way of adoption has no cause for inferiority.

Before you become enthusiastic over pursuing the adoption route there are several factors to consider.

1. Be resolved in your own mind that you do really want and will accept an adopted child. Adoption is not for everyone, and no couple should go on a "guilt trip" because they are not ready to accept an adopted child. A friend of ours who recently underwent a miscarriage after several years of infertility, told us that for her adoption was out. "Being pregnant was such a special feeling," she said, "I just couldn't go any other way to have a baby." She may change her mind, of course, but for now adoption

is not for her, and that is legitimate. There is such tremendous outside pressure on many infertile couples to
have children that some adopt in response to this pressure. That is unfortunate and unfair both to the child and
the couple.

2. Undoubtedly many of you know there is a shortage
of healthy, adoptable babies in America today. What you
may not realize is just how bad the shortage is. When we
adopted John Mark in 1978, the waiting period was approximately two years. When we adopted Sarah in 1982,
the waiting period was approximately four years. In 1984,
for some agencies it was closer to eight! Twenty-five years
ago nine-out-of-ten pregnant, unmarried women who did
not have abortions were electing to have their babies
adopted; today nine-out-of-ten are keeping their babies.

With today's scarcity of adoptable children, you are advised to contact as many agencies as possible. Ask if they
are accepting applications, what their fees are, if there are
any special restrictions, etc. Take care to select the agency
which has the greatest potential for helping you to adopt
a baby in a reasonable amount of time.

3. Adoption is expensive. For some couples the several
thousands of dollars for adoption in addition to the thousands already spent on infertility treatment may be pro-
hibitive. Some agencies take into account the financial
situation of the couple (thankfully, ours did), but others
do not. A few require no fee at all because their expenses
are covered by grants and endowments. On average, one
should expect to pay from $3,000 to $10,000 in adoption
fees.

4. Even though you have struggled through the implications of adoption yourselves, remember that your family and friends may not have reached that point with you.
Initially, those close to you, especially parents, may react
somewhat coolly to the idea that you are pursuing adoption. They may still be very hopeful that you will have a
biological child, even though that hope has been dying in

your own heart. Be patient with any negative reaction. Your family needs time to grow accustomed to the idea of adoption, just as you needed time yourself.

5. Be prepared for the anxiety of waiting.

For us the waiting was the worst. We had been told that we could expect a wait of about two years. Several months before the two years were up we could not stand it anymore so we called the agency to see how we were coming. Guardedly they told us that we could expect a baby "soon." But what did "soon" mean? Tomorrow? Next week? Six months from now? Knowing that a baby is coming via an adoption agency is not the same as having a baby coming via a pregnancy. In a pregnancy there is tangible, objective evidence that a baby is coming and you know when (give or take a few days).

In lieu of anything tangible we made few preparations for the coming of a baby. If it was indeed going to be a matter of months and not days we did not want the constant reminder to make us any more anxious than we already were. What is more, subconsciously we wanted to guard against the vague but uneasy fear that something might go wrong and we would have no baby.

6. After the wait, comes the joy, and it is a shared joy. Earlier it was said that when family and friends learn that you are considering an adoption, you may receive a cool reaction. That still stands. But usually this fades very quickly. Once an adopted child is brought into the home, adoptive parents are often overwhelmed with support! Friends of the adopting couple become almost as excited as the parents. Adopting couples probably receive more baby gifts than those who have a biological child. Church members tend to rejoice enthusiastically with the adopting family.

On the Sunday when we announced in church that we had adopted a baby, one elderly man started clapping wildly. We started receiving gifts from people we hardly knew. For us and many adoptive parents this shared joy becomes a truly great experience.

Do It Yourself

The desperate desire for the privilege of being parents and the critical shortage of adoptable babies have led some couples to pursue unusual and sometimes quasi-legal methods to obtain a baby.

One approach has been termed the "gray market baby."

Typically, it works like this. A woman with an unwanted pregnancy learns about a doctor and/or lawyer in town who has the reputation (gained by word of mouth) of paying all medical costs for labor and delivery (and sometimes prenatal living expenses as well) for any woman who will be willing to give her child up for adoption.[1] At the same time, this doctor/lawyer develops the reputation among infertility circles of having adoptable children available. When prospective adoptive parents come to such a lawyer or doctor, he may be able to supply them with a baby they can legally adopt. Naturally, the fee for this kind of service can be very high! Some discreet checking with infertile friends will probably yield a name of a lawyer or doctor to contact. If you want to follow this method, first check to see if this is legal in your state.

Some couples pursue a more creative and independent approach to obtain a baby. They simply advertise for one. We know of a couple who wrote a letter not only to all the physicians within a 500-mile radius, but also to anyone they had ever met describing their desire for a baby and asking the recipient to contact them if he or she became aware of a mother-to-be who might want to place her child for adoption. It took a lot of effort, but it worked.

1. It is important to note that a woman may not be paid a fee to give up her child. That would involve what are called "black market babies" and this is illegal in every state.

This and other approaches are described in the book called *Beating the Adoption Game* by Cynthia D. Martin (San Diego: Oaktree Publications, 1980).

All of the alternatives to agency adoption which we have described so far fall under the heading of "private adoptions." Personally, we have mixed feelings about the advisability of private adoptions. They can and have worked well for some people, but there can also be significant risks. Foremost among them is the possibility that the birth mother will change her mind at the last moment and decide to keep the child that has been born to her. She may enter the hospital determined that she will not keep the baby, but once she has delivered and held that child in her arms a powerful emotional reaction can develop and suddenly she is not at all sure she wants to part with this beautiful little person to whom she has given birth.

This can be a devastating blow to an infertile couple who had set their hearts on receiving this child into their home. It is equivalent to experiencing a death in the family.

There can also be legal complications. Most adoption agencies have a long history of carefully completing the necessary legal groundwork to ensure that when the adoption is finalized by the court there is virtually no chance of the adoption being revoked later on. Unfortunately, not all doctors and lawyers who are involved in private adoptions are as careful. Recently in a nearby city this caused a heart-rending situation. A couple had received a child into their home through private adoption, but the lawyer had never obtained the proper consent forms from the child's birth parents. About a year after giving up her child for adoption, the birth mother changed her mind, and because of the improper way her consent had been originally obtained, the judge gave her custody of the child. Thankfully these kinds of situations are unusual, but they develop often enough to make us very leery of private adoptions.

International and Hard-to-Place Children

One option many couples are considering is the adoption of a child with physical or mental handicaps. The best source for such children is the Department of Social Services in your state or your state adoption agency.

Children from foreign countries are also available. Korean children are the most prevalent, but there are also children available from countries such as Columbia, Guatemala, the Philippines, and Mexico. Holt's adoption program in Eugene, Oregon, is probably the most widely known agency which specializes in foreign adoption.

Where to Find Help

The first step in locating available adoption agencies is to check the listing of adoption agencies in the Yellow Pages of your phone book. Additional sources may be found by asking your pastor, checking with a hospital social worker, or contacting a local center for unwed mothers. The Salvation Army sponsors such homes in many communities.

You may also write to the following national organizations which will refer you to adoption resources in your area:

North American Center for Adoption
67 Irving Place
N.Y., 10003
(212) 254-7541

National Committee for Adoption
1341 Connecticut Ave., N.W., Suite 326
Washington, D.C. 20036
(This organization also operates a National Adoption
   Hotline - 202-463-7563)

Helpful books that have been written on adoption include:

Adoption—The Grafted Tree, Laurie Wishard and Williams Wishard. (San Francisco: Cragmont Publications, 1979).

Successful Adoption, Jacqueline Horner Plumez. (New York: Harmony Books, 1982).

You're Our Child: A Social/Psychological Approach to Adoption, Jerome Smith and Franklin I. Miroff. (New York: University Press of America, 1981).

If you are interested in adopting internationally, we recommend that you contact the Holt Adoption Agency, P.O. Box 2420, Eugene, Oregon 97402.

We also strongly recommend a subscription to *OURS* magazine (3307 Highway 100 N., Suite 203, Minneapolis, MN 55422). This magazine contains invaluable information on international adoption. There are local chapters of OURS all over the nation through which couples may meet parents who have adopted internationally.

The Child-Free Lifestyle

For some couples adoption is psychologically untenable or perhaps financially impossible. The onus of age has caught up with other couples and adoption agencies no longer find them acceptable. Some infertile couples will remain childless for a variety of reasons.

If you are an infertile couple who faces the very real possiblity of having no children, either biologically or through adoption, please remember: there is nothing wrong with an infertile couple remaining child-free. Do not permit anyone to make you feel guilty because you do not have children. Resist the pressure to adopt or have a baby by some biotechnical means that is objectionable to you. Contrary to popular opinion, God has never indicated that children are necessary for happiness and fulfillment in marriage. Joyce Landorf in her well-known film series, *His Stubborn Love*, put it very pointedly when she said: "In the opening chapters of Genesis God declares, 'A man will leave his father and his mother and be united to his wife and they will become one flesh' and there is a period there." A Christian husband and wife can find fulfillment in each other and in service to the Lord, with or without children.

The childless Christian couple can develop many avenues for Christian service which may not be as easy for couples with children to pursue. They could "adopt" some underprivileged children for their special attention or be "children" to an older person who has no children to care for him or her. A childless couple we know opens their home to children who come into their community to attend the local school for the deaf.

Surely we are not suggesting that a childless couple deny the hurt that being childless may bring. It is never safe or wise to deny real pain and disappointment, but a childless couple must not let the pain dominate. The Christian childless couple must not allow infertility to rob them of the joy God intended them to have in relationship to him and the partner whom he has given.

12

Learning to Live with Infertility

Sylvia

Some metaphors have been used in this book to describe the problem of infertility. It has been spoken of as a "struggle," and a "nightmare." Perhaps the best metaphor, however, is that infertility is a "journey."[1]

Infertility can be thought of as a journey because a journey is something that has a beginning and an end; it is purposeful, not pointless; it implies activity, not passivity.

The Journey

Above all, infertility is an *emotional* journey. Before a couple has completed it, all the emotions known to humans will be experienced.

I would like to take you along on the emotional journey

1. Many of the ideas and concepts in this chapter are based on a speech "Infertility: Emotional Milestones," given by P. Cramer at a Resolve/Serano Symposium: *Insights into Infertility*, on April 25, 1981, at the University of Nebraska, Omaha.

of infertility. Hopefully you will recognize yourself at various emotional mileposts along the way. If so, you will know how far you have come and how far you yet have to travel before you reach the God-given acceptance that every infertile couple needs.

There's nothing wrong

The journey begins in a hazy fog. You have been married for a year or more and no children have come. You may have used the "Pill" for the first few months while you settled in or your husband finished school. But you have been off birth control for some time and nothing has happened. You assumed that you would become pregnant easily because your sister is a "fertile Myrtle" who had three children within five years of marriage.

At the back of your mind you begin to wonder why you haven't become pregnant, but there is no worry. Perhaps if you and your husband were able to get away for a few weekends or you felt rested enough to make love more often. Or. . . .

There's something wrong—now what?

You continue on in the fog until slowly, gradually, it begins to lift and you realize something is wrong. You should have become pregnant by this time. Each month you hope for the best, but each month you are disappointed again. You laugh it off when asked when you are going to start your family. "Why get tied down so early?" you say, "We've got to enjoy life a little first." For all the outward lightness, inwardly you are becoming disturbed. What is wrong?

It is something minor

You are ready for the next leg of your journey. In many ways it is the easiest one of all. The fog has lifted now and you have acknowledged that you have a problem. But you are confident that your carefully selected doctor can help you. The path before you is not steep, the burden on your back is not heavy. You have seen no need to pack a suitcase for your journey, just a light overnight bag is enough. You are convinced that your journey will not be long. There is nothing seriously wrong with you—you have always been healthy. You do not even consider the fact that there is anything wrong with your six-foot-four, 190-pound husband.

Shock

And then suddenly you fall off a cliff that you had not seen. You hit the bottom with a startled jar. Your doctor has discovered that there is something seriously wrong with you, or your husband. You are surprised. "Doctor," you say, "you've got to be kidding." But he is not.

Shock is usually the shortest stop on the journey. Soon you will climb back up the cliff and, though you are shaken, you are unbowed.

Denial and anger

In fact, with renewed energy and determination you plunge ahead down the path, only you may do so blindly. Before you know it, you have climbed a sharp, rocky hill. It is the hill of denial. "The doctor must be wrong in his diagnosis." You convince yourself, "God would never allow us not to have children."

The hill of denial soon becomes the hill of anger. You may become angry at your doctor. "He is so insensitive, so incompetent, so expensive." Your anger may turn on your spouse. "Why can't you come with me to the next doctor's appointment?" Your anger at this stage of the journey can go in almost any direction. You may become angry at yourself: "It's stupid to get so upset about this problem." You may even become angry at God.

Guilt and depression

Anger does not usually last long, and before you know it, you are slipping down into the valley of guilt: "If only

I hadn't used birth control"; "If only I had gone to the doctor sooner"; "If only I had been a better Christian." Much of the guilt may be unrealistic, but at the time you do not recognize it.

At the bottom of the valley you encounter depression. The depression can take many forms. You may simply have a dragged-out feeling or feel unattractive and unloved. You may lose all your desire for sex. You may stop caring about your appearance. For some infertile persons the depression can become very serious.

Weariness and isolation

It is difficult to leave depression completely behind, and you may fall into it periodically again, but in the meantime you continue your journey. You discover now that your journey is much longer than you thought at first. Instead of a short walk, you discover that the road stretches on for miles. The sun is burning hotly now as you walk along the dusty road. You are becoming weary and tired. You endure tests and more tests and still no end is in sight.

The worst part of it may be that you feel so alone. No one else seems to be walking with you. Even your husband (or your wife) may not understand. You pray but there seems to be no answer. When you have dared to share your burden with others, they have responded with platitudes.

Ambivalence

At times you climb the uncertain slopes of ambivalence. You are not sure how you feel. At one moment your longing to have children reaches the point of desperation, at the next you tell yourself you do not care if you ever have them. When your friend comes over with her baby, you alternate between wanting to tear that baby out of her arms and wanting to push that baby away from you and out of your sight.

Sometimes you walk along in the dark. Your doubts become very large. "Why, God? What is your plan for me in all of this?"

An oasis of calm

As you reach the conclusion of this phase of your journey, you may come to what has been called an "oasis of calm." This is a little rest period in your journey. It may come because you give your body a little vacation from all the tests and treatments you have been taking. In any case, it is a much needed respite from the journey. You feel a sense of sadness perhaps that you have not achieved your goal, but it is a calm sadness. In a sense, this oasis of calm is a time of preparation for the emotional work to come. The hardest part of the journey is just ahead.

Grief

The most difficult part of the journey is through the river of grief. You begin this part of your journey either as a result of a doctor's report ("I'm sorry, Mrs. Jones, but I don't think there is much point in continuing treatment.") or your own dawning, gnawing realization that you probably will never have a baby.

There is no body when this time of grief occurs. There is no blue-eyed blond-haired child lying in a casket. No memorial service is held in church. No friends offer you condolences. For it is the death of a dream; it is the death of your hopes and aspirations. It is the death of a child you never had.

During this time of grief, all the emotions you felt before may resurface with a vengeance: anger, denial, guilt, desolation, depression, you name it. You cannot concentrate on your work. You may have difficulty in sleeping. The loss becomes more and more and more real, first in spurts and flashes, and then in a long, unremitting stream.

You may not realize at the time that during this stage of your journey you will accomplish a great deal of emotional work, work that will be so necessary if you are to reach the end of the journey. This duty involves the process of burying that which has been lost. What has been lost to you in your infertility? A son who looks like his Dad, a daughter who looks like you? You begin to bury that dream and you mourn. Were you hoping that you could pass on your mother's crystal chandelier to your daughter someday? You bury that hope and you mourn. Was the feeling of being pregnant an urgent desire on your part? Was breast feeding a hope? You also bury that dream and you mourn.

It is difficult to bury all of your dreams and hopes, and some you may not bury completely, but at least you begin the process.

Recovery

After you have grieved and mourned, you begin the journey again. You are through the worst part of the journey now. You are on the way to recovery. It begins when you start to take positive action and sense a budding interest in the future. All the energy that before had been put into grief you now begin devoting to new projects and new beginnings. The room that you may have been keeping for the baby, you decide to change into a den. You begin to cultivate more intensively whatever is fertile ground in your life such as a talent you have neglected, a career you have put on hold, more education in a field that interests you.

Acceptance and peace

Finally you reach the end of the journey. Now you are home. You have reached a sense of God-given peace and acceptance. Your faith has returned in full force. For a long time you have asked "Why me, God?" but now that question no longer seems important. God has been with you. It is enough. Once again you can read Psalm 106 with a smile on your face instead of tears:

Praise the LORD.
Give thanks to the LORD, for he is good;
His love endures forever.

You regain your basic optimistic outlook on life. Instead of being empty, life resumes its full flavor, full of opportunities for enjoyment and service.

You are open with others and can share your loss without weeping or bitterness. You find it less difficult to love your best friend's baby. You sense the needs of others and begin to see that God is using your infertility to make you more sensitive to their loss and hurts.

Does Every Infertile Person Travel this Journey?

Probably every infertile person travels at least a portion of the road. Not every one, however, makes the journey in exactly the sequence outlined here. For some persons, the journey is not as intense; for others it is more intense. Some go through all the stages of the journey, others do not. Some go forward on the journey and then find themselves going backward temporarily to an earlier point. At least half of those who begin the journey will not complete it because thankfully, they will achieve a pregnancy and childbirth along the way.

For some couples there is the significant problem of becoming stuck at some point along the journey. They do not move on in time to another stage in the journey but rather become mired deep in an emotional impasse.

It may be a stop at the point of depression. Instead of experiencing the mild depression that almost every infertile person feels at one time or other, there is a severe depression. The person becomes unable to function. He or she may even consider suicide. Other persons become stuck at the point of isolation, so much so that a wedge between husband and wife develops and divorce is considered.

If you become hopelessly stuck at one of the above points,

or others as serious, we encourage you to seek help from a professional counselor.

If the emotional impact of the fertility problem is beginning to distort the relationship between husband and wife or their relationships with other people, it would be best to discuss with your doctor the necessity of seeing a counselor. Sensitive counseling by a good psychologist or psychiatrist who is familiar with the problems faced by infertility patients can be of inestimable value. Your infertility specialist should be able to guide you to such a counselor.

The "Old Friend"

Learning to live with infertility means that you will never be able to forget it completely. There will probably always be occasions when infertility will bring a stab of pain.

Recently I had a garage sale and decided to sell all my children's outgrown clothes because I knew I would not need them again. One person who stopped by the sale asked me if I had anything for newborn babies. I had to say "No" to her, and to myself I had to say in a sudden feeling of sadness, "I never had my children when they were that small."

But when the pain returns, it is a dull pain, not intense; it is momentary, not long lasting; it only casts a slight shadow and does not cloud my whole day. A paragraph in Barbara Menning's book says it so well:

My infertility resides in my heart as an old friend. I do not hear from it for weeks at a time, and then, a moment, a thought, a baby announcement or some such thing, and I will feel the tug—maybe even be sad or shed a few tears. And I think, "There's my old friend. It will always be a part of me . . ." (p. 117).

I know that "old friend," but thankfully, I know another friend as well, the Lord Jesus Christ. "I can do everything through him who gives me strength" (Phil. 4:13).

Bibliography

Anderson, J. K. *Genetic engineering.* Grand Rapids: Zondervan, 1982.

Asprooth, E. Infertility awareness and the BBTs. *National Resolve Newsletter,* June 1982, p. 7.

Eareckson, J. & Estes, S. *A step further.* Grand Rapids: Zondervan, 1978.

Geisler, N. I. *Ethics: Alternatives and issues.* Grand Rapids: Zondervan, 1980.

Halverson, K. & Hess, K. M. *The wedded unmother.* Minneapolis: Augsburg Publishing House, 1980.

Howard, J. T. & Schultz, D. *We want to have a baby.* New York: E. P. Dutton, 1979.

Kass, L. R. New beginnings in life. In M. Hamilton (Ed.), *The new genetics and the future of man.* Grand Rapids: Eerdmans, 1972, pp. 15-63.

Menning, B. E. *Infertility: a guide for the childless couple.* Englewood Cliffs, NJ: Prentice Hall, 1977.

Stigger, J. A. *Coping with infertility.* Minneapolis: Augsburg Publishing House, 1983.

Yancey, P. *Where is God when it hurts?* Grand Rapids: Zondervan, 1977.

Suggestions for Further Reading

Along with the books and publications already suggested, you may find the following helpful:

Infertility

Andrews, Lori B. *New Conceptions: A Consumer's Guide to the Newest Infertility Treatments*. New York: St. Martin's Press, 1984.

McGowan, John Yuhas. *Waiting: Hopes and Frustrations of a Childless Couple*. New York: Vantage Press, 1983.

Infertility from a Christian Perspective

Anderson, Ann Kiemel. *Taste of Tears, Touch of God*. New York: Thomas Nelson, 1984.

Love, Vicky. *Childless Is Not Less*. Minneapolis: Bethany House, 1984.

McIlhaney, Joe S. *1250 Health-Care Questions Women Ask*. Grand Rapids: Baker, 1985.

Stigger, Judith A. *Coping with Infertility*. Minneapolis: Augsburg Press, 1983.

Pregnancy Loss

Berezin, Nancy. *After a Loss in Pregnancy*. New York: Simon & Schuster, 1982.

Pizer, Hank & O'Brien. *Coping with a Miscarriage*. New York: Dial Press, 1980.

Vredevelt, Pam W. *Empty Arms: Emotional Support for Those Who Have Suffered Miscarriage or Stillbirth*. Portland: Multnomah Press, 1984. This book is written from a Christian perspective.

Adoption

Johnson, Patricia Irwin, ed. *Perspectives on a Grafted Tree*. Fort Wayne, IN: Perspectives Press.

Krementz, Jill. *How it Feels to Be Adopted*. New York: Knopf, 1982.

Sorosky, Arthur D., M.D., Baron, Annette, MSW, & Pannor, Rueben, MSW. *The Adoption Triangle*. New York: Anchor Press/Doubleday, 1978.

Glossary

adhesion Scar tissue binding together structures of the body that are not ordinarily attached to each other. This may result from surgery, inflammation, or injury.

AID, AIH. *See* artificial insemination.

artificial insemination Instillation of sperm into the vagina or uterus by medical technique rather than by intercourse. Husband's sperm may be used (AIH) or donor's sperm may be used (AID).

basal body temperature (BBT) Body temperature immediately on awakening in the morning, before any daily activity (including getting out of bed) has begun.

biopsy Surgical removal of portions of the body's tissue for microscopic study and diagnosis.

birth-control pills ("the Pill") A pill containing synthetic estrogens and progesterones or only synthetic progesterone. Use of such pills produces an artificial menstrual cycle and prevents the release of the egg from the ovary each month.

centimeter A unit of measurement; .3937 inch; cc—cubic centimeter, there are about 30 cc in a fluid ounce.

cervix The lower part of the uterus that includes the mouth of the uterus. It is about two inches long and one inch wide in an adult.

161

Clomid (clomiphene citrate) A drug commonly used to stimulate ovulation. Serophene is another name for this drug.

conception The union of sperm and ovum, the male and female sex cells, which leads to the development of a new life. It is sometimes called fertilization or impregnation.

contraception A method, device, or substance used to prevent conception.

corpus luteum The structure left in the ovary after ovulation has occurred, formed from the follicle in which the egg developed. The corpus luteum is actually a short-lived gland. After ovulation, it begins producing progesterone and continues this for two weeks, longer if pregnancy occurs.

cyst A sac containing fluid or semisolid material. Some cysts are present in the body as a normal part of its function (i.e., follicle cysts of the ovary which release an egg each month). Some cysts in the body are abnormal growths.

douche A method of cleansing or treating the vagina by irrigating it with water or a water-based preparation.

ejaculation The male orgasm during which seminal fluid (usually containing sperm) is discharged through the penis.

embryo An organism in the earliest stage of development. A human is considered to be an embryo through the first six weeks of life in the uterus.

endometrial biopsy A procedure in which a doctor inserts an instrument into the uterus and scrapes out a portion of the lining of the uterus (endometrium) for evaluation.

endometriosis The lining of the uterus is called the endometrium. When this tissue is present anywhere else in the body, it is called endometriosis. If it is found in the muscular wall of the uterus, it is called adenomyosis.

endometrium The membrane that lines the inner surface of the uterus.

estrogen The primary female sex hormone. A woman's estrogen is principally produced in her ovaries. When the ovaries stop working at menopause, a woman's body will contain very little natural estrogen.

fallopian tubes Structures attached to the upper corner of the uterus on either side. They are about the same shape and size as a normal sized earthworm. The outer ends of the fallopian tubes are open, and it is through them that an egg passes from the ovary to the uterus.

fertile Able to conceive.

fertilization The union of the male sperm and the female egg (ovum).

fiber-optic light This light has made it possible for physicians to brightly illuminate cavities of the body so they can be viewed with small "telescopes." The light bulb is outside the body and is projected at one end of a bundle of flexible glass fibers. This special fiber bundle carries the light to the inside of the body for laparoscopy, hysteroscopy, and other such procedures.

follicle-stimulating hormone (FSH) A female hormone released from the pituitary that is responsible for the development of the egg-containing follicles of the ovaries.

GIFT (gamete intrafallopian transfer) An adaptation of the IVF procedure in which eggs and semen are injected directly into the fallopian tubes by means of a thin tube threaded through an incision made during a laparoscopy or a mini-laparotomy.

gynecology The branch of medicine dealing with diseases of women, particularly those of the reproductive organs and the breasts.

hormone A substance, produced by specialized body tissue called an endocrine gland, that is carried by the blood stream to another part of the body where it has a specific effect.

hysterosalpingogram (HSG) An X-ray procedure in which dye is injected through the cervix into the uterus and out through the fallopian tubes. As the dye is injected, X-rays are taken to facilitate evaluation of a woman's uterus and fallopian tubes.

immunological infertility The presence of sperm antibodies in the male or female which decreases the sperm's ability to fertilize an egg.

infertility A condition in which a couple does not achieve pregnancy after twelve to eighteen months of regular, normal intercourse, or is unable to carry a child to live birth.

intrauterine insemination (IUI) A relatively new technique for treatment of infertility. Washed sperm (from husband or donor) are inserted directly into a woman's uterus.

in vitro (test tube) fertilization (IVF) A technique whereby a woman's egg is taken from her body and placed in a culture dish to which sperm are added. When fertilization has occurred, the embryo is placed in the woman's uterus, where it develops as any normal pregnancy would.

IUI. *See* intrauterine insemination.

laparoscopy An examination that allows the physician to view the female organs and the abdominal cavity with an optical telescope that is passed through a small incision in the abdominal wall (usually through the lower edge of the navel). Some procedures, such as sterilization, laser operations and cutting apart adhesions can be done at laparoscopy.

laparotomy   Any operation in which the abdominal cavity is opened. In infertility treatment this operation is for the purpose of examining or repairing the reproductive organs.

LH.   See luteinizing hormone.

luteal phase   The part of a woman's monthly cycle which lasts from the moment she ovulates (releases an egg) until her menstrual period starts, (usually fourteen days). It is called the luteal phase because, as soon as ovulation occurs, the ovary is left with a small cystic structure, called the corpus luteum, which produces both estrogen and progesterone until menstruation starts.

luteinizing hormone (LH)   A hormone produced by the pituitary that stimulates the ovary to release its egg.

menstruation   The periodic (monthly) flow of blood and debris from her uterus during a woman's reproductive years.

miscarriage   The loss of a pregnancy by a spontaneous abortion.

morphology   The shape and structure of a sperm.

motility   The sperm's ability to move.

obstetrics   The branch of medicine that deals with pregnancy and childbirth.

ovaries   The glands on either side of the uterus which produce eggs and the hormones progesterone and estrogen.

ovulation   The process in which the egg (ovum) is released from the ovary. In sexually mature females, ovulation usually occurs every twenty-eight days, halfway between the menstrual periods. Ovulation usually starts a fourteen-day chain of events that ends with a menstrual period if pregnancy does not occur. *See* luteal phase.

ovum   Egg cell. When fertilized, it is capable of developing into a person similar to its parents in traits that are hereditary, or transmitted by the genes of the chromosomes.

Pap smear   A procedure in which a few cells are scraped from the vagina or cervix and examined for a possible malignancy.

penis   The male organ of copulation. Also contains the urethra, which carries urine from the body.

PK test.   *See* Sims-Huhner test.

post-coital test. *See* Sims-Huhner test.

progesterone A female hormone produced by the ovaries after ovulation.

prolactin The hormone released in large amounts after childbirth, stimulating the glands in the breasts to produce milk. In some women abnormally high prolactin level can inhibit fertility.

reproductive endocrinologist A doctor specializing in the diseases of the reproductive organs, including the associated endocrine glands, as they relate to the problems of infertility.

retrograde ejaculation (reverse ejaculation) An abnormality characterized by the semen entering the bladder instead of going to the tip of the penis. The condition may be caused by diabetes, neurological disease, or prostatic or bladder surgery.

scrotum The sac of skin that holds the male's testicles.

semen The material which is expelled from a man's penis at ejaculation. The largest component of semen is mucus. In the mucus of the semen is contained the sperm, the most "important" element but the smallest in volume.

Sims-Huhner Test (SHT, also called PK or post-coital) A diagnostic procedure used to evaluate the receptivity of a woman's cervical mucus to her husband's sperm. It is normally done a day or two before ovulation and two to four hours after intercourse. It is painless and is much like a routine Pap smear.

sperm The male reproductive cell. *See* semen.

sterility Incapacity to produce children, in either the female or the male.

testicles, testes Two male sex glands which hang outside the body in a sac called the scrotum. They produce sperm and testosterone, the male sex hormone.

testicular biopsy A microscopic examination of a small piece of tissue from the testicles to determine if sperm are being produced. The testicular tissue is obtained by a quarter-inch incision in the scrotum.

testosterone The primary male sex hormone.

tubal pregnancy A form of ectopic pregnancy in which the embryo begins developing in the fallopian tubes. Other forms of ectopic pregnancy are abdominal pregnancies and ovarian pregnancies.

urologist Bladder and kidney specialist. These physicians treat kidney or bladder problems. They also treat men for problems of male infertility.

uterus (womb) Hollow, pear-shaped organ in the female pelvis that carries an unborn child for nine months and from which the menstrual flow comes.

vagina Female genital passage which extends from the vulva to the uterus.

varicocele An accumulation of veins around the testicle that can occasionally result in a man's sperm count or sperm quality being lower than normal, with resulting fertility problems. Such a condition can usually be cured with a minor operation.

vas deferens or "vas" The narrow tube through which sperm travel from the testes of the male to the seminal vesicles.

vasectomy Sterilization surgery on the male accomplished by cutting the vas, the tube that carries the sperm from the testicles to the internal sex organs.